The Adult ADHD & ADD Solution

Discover How to Restore Attention and Reduce Hyperactivity in Just 14 Days. The Complete Guide for Diagnosed Children and Parents

By Julia Kruger

© Copyright 2018 - All rights reserved.

The content contained within this book may not be reproduced, duplicated or transmitted without direct written permission from the author or the publisher.

Under no circumstances will any blame or legal responsibility be held against the publisher, or author, for any damages, reparation, or monetary loss due to the information contained within this book. Either directly or indirectly.

Legal Notice:

This book is copyright protected. This book is only for personal use. You cannot amend, distribute, sell, use, quote or paraphrase any part, or the content within this book, without the consent of the author or publisher.

Disclaimer Notice:

Please note the information contained within this document is for educational and entertainment purposes only. All effort has been executed to present accurate, up to date, and reliable, complete information. No warranties of any kind are declared or implied. Readers acknowledge that the author is not engaging in the rendering of legal, financial, medical or professional advice. The content within this book has been derived from various sources. Please consult a licensed professional before attempting any techniques outlined in this book.

By reading this document, the reader agrees that under no circumstances is the author responsible for any losses, direct or indirect, which are incurred as a result of the use of information contained within this document, including, but not limited to, — errors, omissions, or inaccuracies.

Table of Contents

Chapter 1: What is ADD & ADHD? 6
- Introduction to ADD & ADHD 6
- What Causes ADHD? 7
- Which Groups Are At Risk? 8
- Common Misconceptions about ADHD 16

Chapter 2: Child with ADHD 25
- What Causes ADHD among Kids? 27
- Symptoms of a Child With ADHD 29
- Criteria for Diagnosing ADHD in Kids 30
- Diagnosing ADHD in Kids 31
- Which Other Disorders Accompany ADHD Among Kids? 36

Chapter 3: Attention Deficit Hyperactivity Disorder in Adults 39
- Symptoms of Adult ADHD 40
- The Appearance of ADHD Symptoms Amongst Adults 42
- Diagnosing ADHD in Adults 42
- Couples with ADHD 44

Chapter 4: Medical and Treatment Guidance for ADHD 55
- Medication for ADHD Types 55
- Treatment in Kids 58
- Treatment of ADHD in Adults 69
- How Long Should ADHD Medication be Administered? 71
- Should Patients Consider Psychotherapy? 72
- ADHD Coaching 73
- Can ADHD Be Treated Without Drugs? 74
- Alternative Interventions to Medicines and Therapy 75

 Recommended Food & Supplements to help with ADHD 78
Chapter 5: ADHD and Other Mental Disorders 83
 ADHD With Learning Disabilities in a Child............................. 83
 ADHD with Autism Spectrum Disorder in a Child and an Adult 86
 ADHD With Anxiety 90
 ADHD With Depression 96
 Tips to Overcome Depression With ADHD 100
 ADHD With Bipolar Disorder 101
Conclusion 105
The Mind with Cognitive Behavioral Therapy..................... 106

Congratulations on purchasing The Adult ADHD & ADD Solution, and thank you for doing so!

The following chapters will discuss how to Overcome ADHD as a Parent. The Effects on Marriage and Relationships. Best ways to Parenting kids and teenagers with ADHD. The information found in this book will best explore the diets and treatments in order to Restore Focus and attention.

Thanks again for choosing this book! Every effort was made to ensure it is full of as much useful information as possible.

Please enjoy!

Chapter 1: What is ADD & ADHD?

Introduction to ADD & ADHD

ADHD (attention deficit hyperactivity disorder) is among the most prevalent childhood disorders. This learning disorder was formerly known as ADD (attention deficit disorder) and according to the Center for Disease Control and Prevention, more than 6.4 million children have been diagnosed with it. The disorder has an effect on the behavior, learning ability, and emotions of those who are affected. In as much as ADHD is most prevalent among children, it is also common in adults. Those who are affected by this condition in adulthood always start experiencing its symptoms in childhood.

The rate of ADHD prevalence amongst school-going children is estimated to be 11%. Most cases end up being diagnosed because ADHD typically overlaps other behavioral disorders that weaken individuals' cognitive skills, thus making it difficult for clinicians to categorize whatever they see. It has largely been claimed that ADHD is a modern disorder owing to the fact that it has only been on the rise in recent years.

Pinpointing the rate of ADHD prevalence in all demographics of the population remains a grey area because there are glaring discrepancies among people who are diagnosed with it. The situation is compounded further by the fact that mental health specialists use varying criteria to diagnose the disorder. Besides this, cultural factors pertaining to what should be considered normal behavior varies from one place to another. Behaviors that point towards the positive diagnosis of ADHD in some places could be considered normal in other regions.

What Causes ADHD?

Even though no one can explicitly point out the exact cause of ADHD, it has been proven that various factors play a contributory role. Since ADHD symptoms- inattention, hyperactivity and/or impulsivity affect a child's or adult's ability to get along with others, many people assume that the behavior exhibited by such individuals is as a result of poor discipline, a chaotic upbringing, or even too much TV watching. This is skewed thinking since ADHD traits run in families. Up to half of adults who have ADHD will end up having kids with the disorder. Generally, there are generic traits which get passed down from an ADHD adult to his/her kids. If an adult has ADHD, there's a 50% chance that his/her kids will have it. Likewise, there's a 30% chance of ADHD being present in a younger sibling if an older sibling has it. Nevertheless, the manner in which ADHD is inherited is complex since it cannot be linked to one genetic fault.

Research also indicates that ADHD can be caused by an individual's brain structure and function. There are various possible differences in the brain of individuals who have ADHD and those that do not have the condition. Even so, the exact difference isn't clear. For instance, studies on brain scans have revealed that certain parts of the human brain may be smaller in individuals who have ADHD compared to those who don't have the condition. Likewise, other parts may be abnormally larger. Other studies have also suggested that individuals who have ADHD tend to have an imbalance as far as the level of neurotransmitters in their brain is concerned. In other cases, these neurotransmitters do not function properly. Pregnancy problems are also likely to lead to ADHD. Children who have low birth weight and those who are born prematurely are likely to have ADHD.

Which Groups Are At Risk?

Researchers believe that certain groups are at more risk of having ADHD. This includes babies who are born prematurely before the 37th week of pregnancy, and those who have a low birth weight. Similarly individuals who have epilepsy are at high risk of also having ADHD. Those who have brain injury that occurred either in the womb during pregnancy or after a severe impact on the head later in life are also at a high risk of suffering from ADHD.

Mothers who endure difficult pregnancies are also likely to give birth to kids who are at a high risk of having the disorder. Likewise, kids who have head injuries at the brain's frontal lobe are also at a high risk of being diagnosed with ADHD. Toxins also raise the chances of having ADHD with studies indicating that pregnant mothers who drink alcohol or smoke are at a high risk of giving birth to children with ADHD. Likewise, exposure to PCBs, pesticides, and lead during pregnancy also increases the chances of having ADHD. Such toxins typically interfere with kids' brain development.

Types of ADHD

The Diagnostic and Statistical Manual of Mental Disorders indicates that there are three main types of ADHD. These are:

- Inattentive ADHD
- Hyperactive-Impulsive ADHD
- Combination Type ADHD

People who have ADHD may show signs and symptoms of being consistently inattentive just the same way that they are likely to be more impulsive and hyperactive than their peers of the same age. Some have a combination of inattentive and impulsive behaviors.

The predominantly hyperactive-impulsive ADHD patients do not portray significant inattention. On the other hand, predominantly inattentive ADHD patients do not exhibit notable hyperactive or impulsive behavior. The combination type displays behaviors that relate to both inattentiveness and hyperactivity.

Hyperactivity-Impulsivity ADHD Type

Individuals who have this type of ADHD often experience immense hyperactivity, which makes them want to be always "on the go." You will see a kid dashing around, talking incessantly, or even playing with whatever they come across. Staying still to concentrate on simple tasks is difficult for such individuals since their mind is always wandering. You will see them squirming in their seats or fidgeting with objects within their reach, or just roaming around the room. Hyperactive adults tend to feel internally restless, something that leads them to undertake several tasks at once. If not well managed, they end up failing in all these tasks because none of them tends to be given the attention that it deserves. Other signs of hyperactivity-impulsivity in kids include blurting out answers even before they hear the whole question, and having difficulty taking turns or waiting in line. Children who have the hyperactive-impulsive ADHD type tend to be disruptive to the extent that they make learning difficult, not only for themselves but also for others.

Managing Hyperactivity-Impulsivity ADHD

Handling someone who has hyperactivity-impulsivity ADHD can be difficult because such individuals always seem to have boundless energy. More often than less, those who have this type of ADHD are seen to be overly aggressive and unruly due to the impulsive nature of their actions and social interactions. Even though these individuals can be sensitive to other people's feelings, their good qualities tend to be eclipsed by their relatively poor impulse control and ability to self-regulate.

To manage hyperactivity-impulsivity ADHD among kids, you should put in place impulse control measures. This may include posting classroom routines and rules to let them know what is expected of them. These rules also act as a constant visual reminder of what they should do at all times. Hyperactivity-impulsivity ADHD can also be managed by preparing kids for any transitions. In most cases, kids suffering from this type of ADHD have meltdowns when exposed to transitions in between activities. Warning them prior to making changes to their schedules gives them time to end one activity and embark on the next one.

When handling kids who have hyperactivity-impulsivity ADHD, you should always be prepared for hyperactive behavior and impulsive reactions. Once you know that a situation can set off impulsive reactions, always have a plan to keep the impulses in check. For instance, assigning coaches to kids suffering from this type of ADHD will help them maintain their self-control and stay focused.

Inattentive ADHD

Those who suffer from this type of ADHD typically have a hard time when it comes to keeping their mind focused on one activity. They tend to get bored easily and switch off their minds from whatever is happening around them. When engaging in activities that they enjoy, such kids won't have any trouble paying attention. Nonetheless, focusing on their attention on deliberate action is difficult. It even gets harder for them to complete tasks or learn something new due to lapses in concentration. Needless to say, kids are natural dreamers. It isn't unusual to find a kid staring into space or lost in thought. Failure to complete tasks assigned to them may ultimately lead to frustration for both child and parent. Your kid could be having inattentive ADHD if he/she constantly finds it difficult to focus.

Inattentive ADHD is sometimes referred to as Attentive Deficit Disorder (ADD). Sometimes, this type of ADHD is mistaken for mood or anxiety disorder, especially among adults. In children, it typically gets mistaken for a learning disorder. It is easy to ignore this behavioral disorder and, consequently, kids who are affected seldom get the treatment that they require. In the long run, this may lead to undue shame and apathy, which can last throughout an individual's life.

Children who have the inattention type of ADHD are rarely hyperactive or impulsive. Nonetheless, they have difficulties when it comes to paying attention. In most cases, they will appear confused, "spacey," slow, or lethargic. They also tend to experience difficulties in processing information as accurately and quickly as other kids. When given oral instructions, they find it hard to process what is required of them. As a result, they end up making frequent mistakes.

The American Psychiatric Association has a diagnostic manual, which lists 9 common symptoms of inattentive ADHD. When diagnosing inattentive ADHD, at least 6 of these symptoms ought to be present, and should also be significantly disruptive. This will merit the diagnosis of inattentive ADHD. Kids are deemed to have inattentive ADHD if they:

- often fail to pay close attention to detail, and consequently end up making careless mistakes in their schoolwork and other activities they engage in.

- often get distracted and are thus unable to concentrate on tasks or activities.

- often have trouble when it comes to following instructions. This makes it difficult for them to complete their chores and any other duties that may be allocated to them.

- often find it difficult to organize tasks and activities.

- often avoid undertaking tasks, or are reluctant to partake in tasks that require sustained mental effort.

- tend to lose items such as notebooks, which are needed to complete tasks assigned to them.

- are forgetful when it comes to their schedules.

Dealing with Inattentive ADHD

In the event that your child is diagnosed with inattentive ADHD, all is not lost, since you can still improve his/her ability to concentrate on tasks and activities. Generally, a combination of therapy and medication works best. You can undertake behavioral therapy yourself to mitigate inattentive ADHD. Parenting tactics that can be incorporated when offering behavioral therapy to kids with inattentive ADHD may include setting up a reward system for good behavior, and withholding privileges or taking away rewards in an effort to deal with undesirable behavior. Such methods can be used by teachers, parents, and counselors, to help kids who have inattentive ADHD stay on track.

Since children who suffer from inattentive ADHD are forgetful, you can keep them up to speed with tasks that they are supposed to do by creating to-do lists. These lists could contain household and school chores as examples. Posting the lists in places where the kids can easily see them, will keep them apprised with whatever they are supposed to do. It is also advisable that you break down projects into small tasks. Bite-sizing projects will go a long way in preventing kids from getting bored. Rather than telling them to do their homework, for instance, you can request them to read one chapter of their language book. This makes the task at hand appear less mentally strenuous and will give them the impetus to undertake them.

To enhance the concentration span of kids with inattentive ADHD, you should always give them clear instructions. Whatever instructions that you give to them ought to be simple and easy to decipher. Any complexities are likely to cause such kids to switch off their brains, even before they undertake the task at hand. In addition, you should get them into a routine, since a sense of order goes a long way in helping inattentive ADHD kids stay focused. Following a known routine on a daily basis will let them know what is expected of them. You should similarly endeavor to minimize distractions around inattentive ADHD kids since they tend to snap out of concentration even with the slightest disruption. At home, turn off the TV, computers, and video games when the kids are undertaking a task. Likewise, ask their teachers to move them away from doors or windows at school so that they do not get distracted by activities happening outside the classroom. You should also offer rewards whenever inattentive ADHD kids finish tasks on time. Making them feel appreciated will spur them to be more attentive when undertaking future tasks.

Combination ADHD

Combination type ADHD manifests itself when both hyperactivity-impulsivity and inattention are present. In this case, those affected will have the inability to focus at some point and likewise; they will also be unable to stay still at another point. Most kids experience the combination type of ADHD and this is perhaps why the behavioral disorder is rarely diagnosed and treated during childhood. Most of us think that it is normal for kids to experience bouts of hyperactivity and impulsivity followed by inattention.

When someone exhibits 6 or more symptoms of either inattentive or hyperactivity-impulsivity ADHD, chances are high that he/she could be suffering from combination type ADHD. Therefore, a doctor will look out for symptoms of both inattentiveness and hyperactivity when diagnosing combination type ADHD. The diagnosis of this disorder typically involves undertaking a medical examination to rule out other behavioral disorders, such as anxiety. A medical examination may also involve surveys to establish your child's behavior and interaction with others.

Combination type ADHD treatments involve both medication and therapy to improve the child's attention, besides lowering his/her hyperactivity or impulsivity. Psycho-stimulants may be used to ease common behavioral symptoms of combined ADHD, thus making it easier for kids to focus on their everyday tasks.

The symptoms that kids exude are what help determine the type of ADHD that they are suffering from. Since symptoms exhibited by patients may be caused by a different behavioral disorder, it is advisable that patients undergo a thorough diagnosis to determine the type of ADHD that they are suffering from. ADHD symptoms tend to appear over a long period. More often than less, symptoms of hyperactivity and impulsiveness precede those that characterize inattentive ADHD. Besides this, different ADHD symptoms emerge in different settings. For instance, a kid who cannot sit still or portrays disruptive behavior in school is more likely to be noticed than an inattentive daydreamer within the same setting. Likewise, impulsive kids who typically act before thinking are said to have discipline issues while those who exhibit passive behavior are likely to be seen as being merely unmotivated or lazy.

Such prognosis is wrong, considering the fact that both sets of kids show behaviors that point towards different types of ADHD. Generally, all kids sometimes get restless, just the same way that they act without thinking at times. Likewise, kids sometimes daydream their time away. Exhibiting any of these signs alone doesn't show that a kid has ADHD. That can only be the case if a child's distractibility, poor concentration, hyperactivity, or impulsivity, begins to affect their school performance, social relationships, and overall behavior. When this happens, ADHD may be suspected. Since ADHD symptoms vary from one setting to another, diagnosing the condition, therefore, isn't easy.

Test Your Type of ADHD

Just like it is the case with most behavioral disorders, there is no single test that can be exclusively used to diagnose ADHD in both kids and adults. A combination of psychological tests and rating scales to determine the symptoms of ADHD will help you determine whether or not you are affected by the condition. When testing for your type of ADHD, you should first know the symptoms of each. If you exhibit at least six symptoms of hyperactivity-impulsivity, you could have this type of ADHD. Likewise, you could have the inattentive type of ADHD if you have at least six symptoms that characterize the disorder. If you have combination type ADHD, you will certainly exhibit symptoms of both hyperactivity-impulsivity and inattentiveness.

Common Misconceptions about ADHD

A lot of myths and misconceptions about ADHD exist in the public domain. Much of the misinformation about ADHD pertains to its causes, diagnosis, and treatment. The following are some of these common myths.

Only Kids can have ADHD

This is perhaps the most peddled misconception as far as ADHD is concerned. Contrary to what many people think, ADHD affects both children and adults. The misconception that only kids can be affected by this behavioral disorder, is attributed to the fact that its symptoms ought to be exhibited by the age of 7 years so that the criteria for diagnosis is met. A large number of those who are affected remain undiagnosed until they reach adulthood. In some cases, ADHD is diagnosed in adults only after diagnosis has been made on their own kids.

A number of adults only recognize that they have ADHD traits after learning more about it. Such a realization may lead you to reflect on your own childhood and recall whatever struggles you had in school and problems with inattention, that weren't ever treated. You should keep in mind that up to 70% of kids who have ADHD will continue exhibiting symptoms of the conditions up to the time they reach adulthood.

Hyperactive behaviors that are common in children who have ADHD may decrease as they age, but nonetheless, ADHD symptoms, such as inattention, restlessness, and distractibility, may persist into adulthood. If left untreated, adult ADHD often leads to chronic problems at work and in social relationships. It can lead to more serious issues such as depression, anxiety, and substance abuse.

ADHD Only Exists in Your Head

Hypothetically, ADHD is a mental issue, because certain brain regions of patients who have the disorder fail to synchronize properly. This has led many to believe that people only use ADHD as a justification for not focusing on completing their tasks. Nonetheless, this isn't the case. It goes without saying that the brains of individuals with ADHD work differently from those of people who do not have the condition. In the former, the medial prefrontal cortex and the posterior cingulate cortex don't match up, thus leading to concentration issues. This alone proves that ADHD isn't just a typical mental issue used as an excuse for lack of focus when undertaking tasks.

ADHD Signifies Laziness and Lack of Motivation

This misconception is a typical response to behaviors exhibited by kids struggling with inattentive ADHD. In most cases, such kids are seen to be lazy and unmotivated because we fail to look at the underlying cause of their lethargic behavior. Your kid could be finding it difficult to undertake tasks that require continued mental exertion, not because he/she is lazy, but due to ADHD. Therefore, this disorder should not be used as an excuse to label someone as lazy or unmotivated. Besides this, ADHD has nothing to do with an individual's intellectual ability. Plenty of individuals who struggle with the condition are extremely creative and sharp; they only work in a manner that is different from others.

ADHD is Over-Diagnosed

This misconception is informed by the fact that the number of diagnosed ADHD cases has been on the rise in the recent past. Although the number of reported ADHD diagnoses has increased significantly, it shouldn't be misconstrued to mean that the condition is over-diagnosed. It simply means that many people are waking up to the realization that ADHD is real. Consequently, more people are seeking diagnosis and treatment thus the increase in reported cases.

You Must be Hyperactive to Have ADHD

This misconception perhaps stems from the "hyperactive" part of the disorder's title Many people think that you only need to be hyperactive for you to have ADHD. Such individuals tend to forget that predominant inattentiveness and a combination of inattentiveness and hyperactivity also signify someone as having ADHD. Since the inattentive type of ADHD is less disruptive, you may think that those affected do not suffer from ADHD. Likewise, having trouble focusing on tasks doesn't automatically mean that you have ADHD.

If You Can Concentrate on Some Tasks, You Do Not Have ADHD

The fact that ADHD is largely an "attention deficit" disorder makes it quite confusing when you see someone with it concentrating intently on a task. It seems even more fitting to describe the disorder as a condition that forces individuals to have trouble regulating their attention. In as much as those who are affected by ADHD have significant problems focusing their attention on completing tasks, they still maintain the ability to focus on activities that are stimulating. This is known as hyperfocus.

Medicine Can Treat ADHD

Medications, including stimulants and non-stimulants, play an important role in curbing common ADHD symptoms. A combination of treatment goes a long way in manage ADHD. Nonetheless, medicines shouldn't be used in isolation, since behavioral therapy and DIY strategies, such as leaving reminders and notes around the house to keep you up to speed with tasks that you are supposed to undertake, play an important part in minimizing the effects of ADHD.

In as much as medication is the most effective intervention against ADHD, it isn't the only intervention that works. Combining medication with cognitive and behavioral therapy will help quell the symptoms of ADHD. It is important for parents whose kids have ADHD to seek other alternatives which can help manage symptoms of the conditions.

Contrary to public perception, medications used in ADHD management do not cure the condition. Their purpose is to help control common ADHD symptoms. ADHD is a chronic behavioral disorder that doesn't go away it is only the symptoms that may lessen or change over time. Developing organizing and coping strategies will help manage and control the symptoms of ADHD.

ADHD Is not a Real Medical Condition

This is one of the most common ADHD myths that you will find out there. Many argue that ADHD is just a behavioral condition and not a medical condition. According to the [National Center for Disease Control](#) and the [American Psychiatric Association](#), ADHD is a medical condition. It is hereditary in nature since one out of every four people who have ADHD has a parent who also has the condition. Similarly, imaging studies have shown that there is a difference in the brain development of kids who have ADHD and kids who do not have the condition.

ADHD Results from Bad Parenting

This is another common ADHD myth in the public domain. Generally, individuals who have ADHD tend to exhibit antisocial behavior. Many people end up believing that the cause of this behavior is bad parenting. It common for people to attribute inappropriate comments or constant fidgeting among individuals with ADHD, to poor parenting. Unbeknown to them, these are some of the standouts signs of ADHD and have nothing to do with parenting.

ADHD Kids Can Concentrate if they Try Harder to Pay Attention

Kids and adults who have ADHD often struggle to pay attention. Many people believe that the lack of attention is deliberate and that those with ADHD can concentrate if only they try or learn to pay attention. What many people don't know is the fact that ADHD patients often try as hard as "normal people" to pay attention. Telling individuals who have ADHD to focus is akin to asking a short-sighted person to look farther without wearing glasses.

Research indicates that there is a difference in the pathways of the brains kids and adults with ADHD. Generally, these pathways take longer to develop or may function less efficiently and therefore, such individuals end up experiencing concentration lapses.

ADHD Individuals Cannot Focus

Some people who tend to get easily distracted often have trouble shifting their attention from tasks that they enjoy the most. For instance, a child who is watching cartoons or playing with toys can be hyper-focused on that activity. This doesn't necessarily mean that such a child can pay better attention to tasks than kids who have ADHD. It's only a matter of interest in whatever activity that they are engaged in rather than an issue of hyperfocus or lack of focus.

Everyone who has ADHD is Hyperactive

It has long been believed that hyperactivity is the only symptom of ADHD. This is a flawed line of thought since not everyone who is hyperactive has ADHD. Likewise, not everyone who has ADHD is hyperactive. This highlights the importance of understanding the different ADHD types before making an assessment of an individual's behavior.

ADHD Only Affects Males

Needless to say, boys are at a higher risk of having ADHD compared to girls. However, this has been construed to mean that ADHD only affects males. Generally, girls can also have ADHD only that it tends to be overlooked and thus remains undiagnosed. From a young age, society thinks it's normal for boys to be hyperactive, and girls to be less active. This could perhaps explain why many people have been led to believe that ADHD is a male affair. Attention issues tend to be different in boys than girls. Often, girls who have ADHD tend to have less difficulty when it comes to impulse and hyperactivity control. They are likely to seem more "day-dreamy" and out of touch with things happening around them.

As far as ADHD is concerned, girls generally tend to have less trouble than boys especially with hyperactivity. Nonetheless, this doesn't mean that they never experience hyperactivity. Instead, it will look different in them compared to boys. Girls often come across as being overly emotional or hypersensitive. Parents and teachers may notice them barging into conversations or even being a little more chatty than normal girls. For this reason, girls with ADHD are likely to fly under the radar.

ADHD is a Learning Disability

In as much as ADHD hinders the ability to pay attention and learn, it is a behavioral disorder and not a learning disability. It is only the main symptoms of ADHD that impact individuals' overall ability and capacity to learn. It goes without saying that kids can't do well in school or in their social interactions if they lack the ability to focus.

While ADHD only affects focus, learning disabilities tend to affect specific skills such as solving mathematical quizzes. The popularity of the myth that ADHD is a learning disability is attributed to the fact that most learning disabilities occur in comorbidity with ADHD. Similarly, the fact that ADHD is not a learning disability shouldn't mean that kids can't receive help. Devising an Individualized Educational Program can go a long way in helping ADHD kids learn just like other kids.

Kids With ADHD Will Eventually Outgrow It

ADHD is a lifelong disease, which nobody can outgrow. Many people tend to believe that they can overcome the condition as they grow older. Even though some of the symptoms of ADHD tend to change or disappear altogether as one grows older, it doesn't mean that the condition has disappeared.

As one grows older, he/she is likely to learn ways of managing ADHD symptoms. Many people look at this and conclude that the condition has been overcome. Those who have ADHD during childhood will continue having symptoms throughout their adolescence and adulthood. It is only that some of the symptoms may be subdued.

Chapter 2: Child with ADHD

This behavioral disorder is more common in kids than adults, thus making it necessary for parents to recognize the symptoms of ADHD. This will go a long way in helping them manage the condition in case their kids are affected. It is totally normal for kids to occasionally daydream in class, act impulsively, fidget at the dinner table, or even forget about their homework. What many parents do not understand is that the underlying cause of such behavior could be much deeper than what meets the eye. Impulsivity, hyperactivity, and inattention are some of the most notable signs of ADHD.

We have all encountered kids who cannot stay still, those who don't follow instructions, and those who always seem to be daydreaming. More often than less, such kids are deemed to be troublemakers, lazy, or undisciplined. The behaviors that such kids have are a pointer that they could be suffering from ADHD. Typically, ADHD symptoms in kids appear before they reach seven years. Nonetheless, the unpredictable nature of kids often makes it difficult to distinguish between those who are "normal" from those who are affected by attention deficit hyperactivity disorder.

It is generally advisable that you take a close look at your kid if he/she starts exhibiting a number of ADHD symptoms across different situations when playing, at home, and in school. It is only after you have understood the exact ADHD issue that your kid is struggling with, that you can work out a creative solution for remedying the disorder.

The stereotypical ADHD patients is an 8-year old kid who has the tendency to jump off from high points dangerously, or never even remembers to raise his/her hand while in class. In reality, only a few people who have ADHD fit this description.

Generally, kids who have the tendency to bounce off chairs or prank their playmates are usually the first ones to be evaluated for ADHD and to be diagnosed. On the other hand, those that have the tendency to have the tendency to wander off while in class often fly off the radar.

The National Institute of Mental Health points out that most inattention symptoms are less likely to be pinpointed by parents, medical professionals, and teachers. As a result, those who suffer from inattention ADHD rarely receive the treatment that they need. These kids often exhibit symptoms of academic frustration, undue shame due to poor academic and social performance, and apathy. These may last throughout their lifetime.

Often, inattention ADHD is regarded as spacey and apathetic behavior among kids, and mood disorders among adults. Individuals who suffer from inattention ADHD tend to lose focus when engaging in mentally exerting tasks. They are also forgetful, and have trouble listening. Kids who have inattention ADHD may rush through quizzes while missing questions whose answers they know, or they may even skip whole sections in their haste. This habit may persist until adulthood whereby adults who have ADHD often fail to proofread documents carefully at work. This way, they end up attracting unwanted embarrassment and attention.

Kids who have inattention ADHD similarly have a shorter attention span compared to other kids. They will submit unfinished classwork, incomplete reading assignments, or do house chores halfway. As they grow older and transition into adulthood, they will despise long work meetings more than their "normal" colleagues do. To sustain their attention during meetings, you will find them sipping coffee, chewing gum or standing up during meetings. In addition, they have poor listening skills besides lacking the ability to follow up on tasks.

What Causes ADHD among Kids?

Needless to say, one of the first questions that you will ask yourself when one of your kids has been diagnosed with ADHD is, "what went wrong?" In as much as we cannot explicitly pinpoint one factor that leads to ADHD, research indicates that the disorder is caused by a myriad of factors. There is little evidence to suggest that ADHD arises purely from either child-rearing methods or social factors. Most of the substantiated causes tend to fall within the realm of genetics and neurobiology. Nonetheless, this shouldn't mean that environmental factors cannot influence the severity of ADHD.

Parents need to focus on finding the best ways of helping their kids cope with ADHD, rather than trying to establish what caused the disorder in the first place. Scientists are still attempting to establish what really causes ADHD in an effort to find better ways of treating and even preventing the condition. They are similarly seeking to prove that ADHD doesn't result from the home environment but rather from biological factors. Such knowledge will relieve parents of the guilt that typically sets in once kids are diagnosed with ADHD.

Here are some of the causes of ADHD.

Environmental Factors

Research indicates that there's a link between cigarette smoking and alcohol consumption during pregnancy, and the occurrence of ADHD in the offspring. As a precaution, pregnant mothers are advised to refrain from cigarettes and alcohol use. A high lead level is another environmental factor that increases the risk of ADHD among kids. Despite the fact that lead isn't allowed in paint, it is still present in older buildings. When pre-school kids are exposed to chemical agents like lead, the risk of ADHD increases.

Brain Injury

One of the earliest theories that were advanced by scientists is that, just like other attention disorders; brain injury greatly contributes to ADHD. Notably, children who have been involved in accidents that eventually led to brain injury tend to have ADHD-like behaviors, including inattention. Nevertheless, it has been established that only an insignificant percentage of kids who have ADHD have suffered traumatic brain injuries in their lives.

Sugar and Food Additives

It has long been suggested that most attention disorders, including ADHD, are caused by the consumption of food additives and refined sugars. Other researchers claim that most ADHD symptoms are exacerbated by food additives and sugar. The National Institutes of Health even held a scientific conference to find consensus on this issue. Ultimately, it was established that diet restrictions only helped a paltry 5% of kids who have ADHD; most of them being young, pre-school children with food allergies.

Genetic Causes

Generally, most attention disorders run in families. Therefore, there is a possibility that ADHD is genetically-transmitted. Research indicates that up to 25% of close family members of kids who have ADHD also have the condition. On the flipside, the rate is only 5% in the general population. Studies among twins also show that there is a notable genetic influence in ADHD. There are ongoing studies that aim to pinpoint the exact genes that cause kids to be vulnerable to ADHD. In line with this, the Attention Deficit Hyperactivity Disorder Molecular Genetics Network was established to act as a platform for researchers to share findings pertaining to possible genetic influences as far as this behavioral disorder is concerned.

Symptoms of a Child With ADHD

When you think of ADHD in kids, what probably comes to mind is a picture of a beyond-control kid who is impulsive and disruptive to everything around them. Nevertheless, this isn't the only behavior that ADHD kids portray. Likewise, kids who always seem docile and uninterested in whatever is happening around them are not lazy or stupid.

ADHD is in kids is akin to a three-lane highway. Some kids who have the disorder will be hyperactive and impulsive at all times. You will see them bouncing off walls, fidgeting with things around them, and generally wanting to engage their seemingly endless energy in physical activities. Such kids similarly react to situations impulsively and will blurt out responses without taking a moment to think. Most times, these kids are seen to be rash, ill-disciplined, and generally unmanaged.

On the other hand, some kids who have ADHD will always seem to be inattentive and detached from events around them. You will find such kids staring blankly into space while in class, with their attention miles away. They hardly engage in social activities and they also find it difficult to complete tasks that are mentally draining. They also find it difficult to shift their attention from one activity to the next.

Inattentive ADHD kids are typically regarded to be lazy and uninterested. Other kids have a unique character that combines hyperactivity and impulsivity with inattentiveness. Kids that show these signs will be hyperactive and impulsive at one point and reclusive at some other point. When interacting with such kids, most of us may end up thinking that they are simply moody and unpredictable.

Criteria for Diagnosing ADHD in Kids

It is important to keep in mind that not every kid who is hyperactive, overly impulsive, or inattentive, is suffering from ADHD. Sometimes, kids simply blurt out things that they didn't mean to say in the first place. Likewise, they are sometimes forgetful and disorganized and even jump from one unfinished task to another. Exhibiting such behaviors doesn't necessarily mean that they have ADHD. Every kid shows these symptoms at some point in their lives. Diagnosing ADHD requires that these symptoms must have been demonstrated over a long time. The behaviors ought to have appeared early in a kids' life (before the age of 7 years), and must have been exhibited for more than 6 months. The behaviors must also have caused a notable handicap in more than two areas of a kid's life, such as in the learning environment and in social settings.

If a kid exhibits some ADHD-related symptoms, yet his/her schoolwork or social interactions are not affected, it would be wrong to diagnose that kid as having ADHD. Besides this, a kid who seems to be overly hyperactive in class, yet functions well elsewhere, can't receive an ADHD diagnosis. To establish whether kids have ADHD, specialists often ask several critical questions; are the behaviors exhibited by a kid excessive? Are they pervasive and long-term? Do they occur in only one specific place or in several settings? In addition, specialists also need to establish whether the behaviors in question occur more frequently in a kid than in other children of the same age. This will help assess whether the behaviors are a continuous problem or simply responses to temporary solutions.

When diagnosing ADHD in kids, their behavioral pattern is typically compared to a specified set of criteria. ADHD-related characteristics are thereafter listed in the DSM-IV-TR (Diagnostic and Statistical Manual of Mental Disorders). This is a manual published by the American Psychiatric Association to provide a common language and standardized criteria for classifying mental disorders.

Diagnosing ADHD in Kids

Most parents notice signs of hyperactivity, impulsivity, and inattention in their kids before they start schooling. Your pre-school kid could have ADHD if he/she loses interest when playing games or watching TV, or even seemingly randomly lose control.

Kids have different personalities, energy levels, and temperaments. They also mature at different rates. Therefore it is advisable to get a behavioral expert's opinion to determine the behavior that is appropriate for your kids at their age. If you suspect that your child has ADHD, you can ask a child psychologist or psychiatrist to either confirm or dispel your fears. Keep in mind that kids often exhibit unusually exuberant and immature behavior and, therefore, you shouldn't hastily conclude that yours has ADHD without having him/her diagnosed by a specialist.

In most cases, ADHD in kids is usually suspected by parents but, nonetheless, remains ignored until they start having problems in school or in their social interactions. Given the fact that the condition tends to mostly affect kids' functioning at school, it is common for teachers to be the first ones to suspect its presence. Once teachers recognize that a kid in their class exhibits prolonged inattentiveness or hyperactivity, it is advisable that they point it out to parents so that ADHD diagnosis and subsequent treatment is undertaken. Since teachers spend time with lots of kids, it is easy for them to know how "normal" kids behave within the class environment. They similarly know how "abnormal" kids behave. Therefore, they are in the best position to inform you whether your kid exhibits prolonged strange behavior in class.

A kid can only be diagnosed with ADHD if he/she exhibits more than six of the nine ADHD symptoms. Similarly, the symptoms must have been observed for more than six months and in more than two settings. It must also be proved that the symptoms are adversely affecting the behavior of that kid. Some of these symptoms must also have been observed before the age of 12.

Who Should Diagnose ADHD in Kids?

Many parents do not know who they should turn to once they suspect ADHD in the kids. Ideally, ADHD diagnosis should be made by child psychologists/psychiatrists, behavioral neurologists, or behavioral/development pediatricians. Clinical social workers can also diagnose ADHD, especially those who have handled similar cases in the past.

Several specialists are qualified to both diagnose and treat the symptoms of ADHD. These specialists can undertake the assessment themselves, or they can serve family members with questionnaires to determine the kids' behavior. Regardless of a specialists' area of expertise, his/her first task should be gathering information that will help rule out various other possible reasons for the kids' behavior.

Possible causes of ADHD-like behavior among kids may include:

- sudden changes in their lives such as their parents' divorce
- unnoticed disorders, such as seizures, including temporal lobe or petit mal seizures
- mental disorders that affect the brain functionality of kids
- middle ear infection, which leads to intermittent hearing problems
- anxiety or depression
- underachievement caused by common learning disabilities

The above mentioned are some of the ADHD-like symptoms that lead parents to suspect that their kids could be suffering from the behavioral disorder. When diagnosing ADHD, these symptoms ought to be ruled out for the diagnosis to be accurate. Ruling out such symptoms when diagnosing ADHD may involve going through a kid's medical and school records. Once it is determined that the kid isn't suffering from any of these conditions, specialists should gather information pertaining to a child's ongoing behavior. This will help them compare their behavior with diagnostic criteria and symptoms that are listed in the DSM-IV-TR. Talking to the child or even observing them in their learning environment and other social settings can go a long way in helping specialists gauge their ongoing behavior.

Diagnosing ADHD in kids should also involve asking teachers about their observations pertaining to the young ones' behavior. These observations should be noted down on standard evaluation forms, which are typically referred to as behavior rating scales. These scales help compare a kid's behavior with that of other children of the same age. Even though rating scales are sometimes overly subjective, they give teachers a valid and reliable measure for determining the long-term behavior of kids under their care.

During diagnosis, specialists can contact anyone who knows the affected kids well, including family members, coaches, and babysitters. Such individuals may be asked to describe the kids' behavior in various situations. In addition, they might also be required to fill out questionnaires or rating scales so that the specialists can determine how frequent and severe the behaviors are.

When diagnosing ADHD among children, their mental health and social adjustment are the main pillars of the assessment.

Besides this, learning achievement and intelligence tests may also be given to determine whether the kids have a learning difficulty.

When looking at the results of various information sources, specialists often pay more attention to the kids' behavior in situations that demand a high degree of self-control. This may include noisy and unstructured circumstances, such as parties and activities that require sustained mental effort; examples can be playing board games or working out mathematical problems.

During ADHD diagnosis, kids' behavior and interaction during free play or when they are given individual attention is usually given less importance. In such circumstances, most children who have ADHD tend to control their behavior and even perform better than when they are in restrictive situations.

After the behavior of kids, who are suspected of having ADHD, has been evaluated over time, specialists often put together a profile that summarizes the observations made over the course of the evaluation. This profile helps the specialists pinpoint ADHD-like behaviors, which are listed in the most recent DSM (Diagnostic and Statistical Manual). A profile similarly helps specialists to determine how frequently these behaviors are exhibited by a kid, whether or not they are periodic in nature, and how long the behaviors are exhibited in each instance. If a kid has any other problems that are related to ADHD, they will also be captured in the profile. Ultimately, the profile will help a specialist determine whether a kid's hyperactivity-impulsivity, inattention, or both, is significant and longstanding. If so, it can be correctly concluded that the kid has ADHD.

A correct diagnosis of ADHD will go a long way in resolving the confusion surrounding a kid's learning problems. It similarly provides the correct information as to what exactly is "wrong" with a kid, and what needs to be done to mitigate the symptoms of the disorder. Thereafter, therapy and medication can be recommended. The kid's family members will also be given educational material about managing ADHD.

Which Other Disorders Accompany ADHD Among Kids?

Learning Disabilities

A significant number of kids with ADHD (30-40%) tend to have specific learning disabilities. In pre-school kids, these learning disabilities are manifested by difficulties in understanding certain words or sounds, and even difficulties in expressing oneself clearly. In school-going children, ADHD-related learning difficulties are typically manifested by spelling or reading disabilities, arithmetic disorders, and writing disorders. Dyslexia, a common type of reading disorder is also quite widespread among children who have ADHD. Even though reading disabilities are common with kids who have ADHD, up to 8% of elementary school kids experience reading difficulties at some point. However, this shouldn't suggest that they also have ADHD.

Tourette Syndrome

An insignificant percentage of kids with ADHD also have Tourette Syndrome. This neurological disorder is characterized by repetitive mannerisms and nervous tics. This may include facial twitches, grimacing, and eye blinks. Others have the tendency to frequently clear their throats, sniff, bark out words, or snort. Behaviors that are related to Tourette Syndrome can easily be treated using medication. Even though very few kids are affected by this disorder, a significant number of those who have it also have ADHD.

Oppositional Defiant Disorder

Up to 50% of kids with ADHD also have oppositional defiant disorder (ODD). This disorder is characterized by non-compliant, defiant, stubborn, and sometimes belligerent behavior among kids. Children who suffer from this disorder tend to experience incessant outbursts of temper and are generally disobedient and argumentative. ODD affects children suffering from hyperactive-impulsivity, inattentive, and combined ADHD types.

Conduct Disorder

Between 20 to 40% of children with ADHD end up developing conduct disorder (CD). This disorder is basically a more serious and complex form of antisocial behavior. Children who have the disorder tend to have antisocial mannerisms such as lying, stealing, bullying others, or fighting. This puts them at risk of falling foul with the law or being aggressive towards everyone around them. As they get older, children who have conduct disorder are at a great risk of drug and substance use.

Anxiety and Depression

Some kids who have ADHD struggle with co-occurring depression and anxiety. Such kids will be in a better position to handle some of the symptoms that accompany ADHD if the anxiety and depression is detected early and treated. Likewise, if ADHD is effectively treated, depression and anxiety among kids is also likely to reduce significantly. This makes it easier for them to handle academic tasks and any other duties that they are asked to perform.

Bipolar Disorder

It is difficult to distinguish between ADHD and bipolar disorder among kids since both conditions have similar symptoms. In its purest form, bipolar disorder is typified by mood swings between periods of extreme highs and lows. Nonetheless, bipolar in children is often a somewhat chronic mood deregulation characterized by a mix of elation, irritability, and depression. Besides this, there are certain symptoms that are present in kids suffering from both bipolar disorder and ADHD, including a decreased need for sleep and high energy levels. Of the main symptoms that are present in kids with bipolar disorder from those with ADHD, grandiosity and elated mood are the distinguishing characteristics.

Chapter 3: Attention Deficit Hyperactivity Disorder in Adults

ADHD among children is so publicized to the extent that not many people know that the disorder also affects adults. What many people don't know is the fact that all kids who have ADHD will still have it in their adult years. Research indicates that up to 70% of children who have ADHD will exhibit symptoms of the disorder during their adult years.

The first study conducted on grown-ups who had never been diagnosed with ADHD during their childhood but showed symptoms of the disorder as adults, was conducted by David Wood, Paul Wender, and Frederick Reimherr. The symptomatic adults were diagnosed with ADHD retrospectively after the researchers interviewed their parents. Ultimately, the trio came up with the Utah criteria, which is a clinical framework for diagnosing adults with ADHD. Generally, the diagnosis of adult ADHD involves evaluating the history of patients, and assessing it against current ADHD-like behaviors. At the moment, there are other diagnostic evaluations for determining the presence of adult ADHD. These include the use of the widely-popular Conners Comprehensive Behavior Rating Scale (Conners CBRS) and the Brown ADD Scales.

It's extremely common for adults who have ADHD to not realize that they have the disorder in the fact place. In cases whereby the disorder was diagnosed and treated in childhood, most adults end up believing that it was fully mitigated and, therefore, it doesn't affect them in adulthood. Whichever the case, adults who have ADHD often feel it is just impossible for them to get organized or even stick to one job for a substantial period. Others even find it difficult to stick to schedules or even keep an appointment. Everyday tasks such as waking up on time, getting to work early, or staying productive at work can be significant challenges to adults who have ADHD.

Symptoms of Adult ADHD

ADHD in adults manifests itself in various ways. Just like with children, adult ADHD can be in the form of hyperactivity and impulsivity, inattention, or a combination of the two. It should be noted that while it isn't difficult to spot ADHD in children, it is hard to in adults. This is attributed to the fact that adults tend to have subtle symptoms, which are hard to spot. This explains why, in most cases, adults struggle with the disorder without knowing that they have it. They fail to recognize that most of the problems that they face in their lives, including staying organized or arriving for meetings on time, relate to ADHD.

Hyperactivity-Impulsivity Symptoms in Adults

If you have the tendency of fidgeting, squirming in your seat, tapping your hands and feet, you probably have adult ADHD. Those who leave their seats even when they are required to remain seated, especially within the workplace setting, could also have ADHD. The disorder is also manifested in instances when you find yourself running where it is inappropriate, or you find it difficult to take part in leisure activities quietly and without feeling restless.

Adults who suffer from the hypersensitive-impulsive type of

ADHD sometimes act as if they are "on the go" or they are being driven by an underlying force. This makes it difficult for them to remain still for extended periods of time, such as when in meetings and restaurants. The tendency to talk excessively while often blurting out answers even before questions have been fully asked could be a sign that an adult it battling with hypersensitive-impulsive ADHD. Such individuals tend to complete other people's sentences, and find it hard to wait for their turn when carrying out conversations. They also tend to intrude into activities and take over from others without seeking permission.

Inattentive ADHD Symptoms in Adults

Adults who find it hard to organize tasks and activities, manage time, and meet deadlines, may also have inattentive ADHD. Besides this, the tendency to avoid, dislike, or show reluctance towards participation in tasks that require concerted or sustained mental effort, points towards inattentive ADHD. This form of ADHD is also manifested in adults who often lose items such as work tools, keys, wallet, important documents, mobile phones, and eyeglasses, and those who easily get distracted when undertaking important things by unrelated thoughts. Forgetfulness in daily tasks such as running errands, paying bills, and returning calls also is a manifestation of inattentive ADHD.

Some adults who suffer from inattentive ADHD may seem not to be carefully listening even when they are spoken to directly. Their minds may be elsewhere even in instances where there seems to be no obvious distraction. Besides this, they often fail to follow through any instructions given to them or duties that they are allocated. Even in instances when they start tasks, they will lose focus quickly or easily get sidetracked.

The Appearance of ADHD Symptoms Amongst Adults

Generally, ADHD among adults appears in different settings. Adults can get affected by ADHD at home, at work, in social situations, or anywhere else. For a positive diagnosis of the behavioral disorder to be made, the aforementioned symptoms ought to be present in more than one setting. Besides this, the symptoms ought to occur more often. ADHD may also appear differently among adults. There must also be evidence that the ADHD symptoms that an adult portrayed interfered with his/her work, academic, and social functions. The symptoms should also not be due to a different mental or behavioral disorder.

Since the condition is a lifelong disorder, which is less noticeable in adults than in kids, many people tend to think that it is less serious during adulthood. What you may not know is the fact that during adulthood, you are vested with more responsibilities and, therefore, any mistake that you make as a result of ADHD is likely to have greater consequences to you and others. For this reason, diagnosing and treating ADHD in adults is just as important as diagnosing and treating it in children.

Diagnosing ADHD in Adults

It isn't easy to diagnose ADHD in adults. Whenever children get diagnosed with ADHD, in most cases parents tend to remember that they may have had the same symptoms during their childhood. This makes them understand some of the behaviors and traits such as restlessness, impulsivity, and distractibility, which are giving their kids problems. Likewise, some adults often discover that they have ADHD after they seek professional help for mental disorders such as anxiety or depression, only to discover that the root of their emotional disorder is ADHD.

For adults to be diagnosed with ADHD, they must have ADHD-like symptoms that started in childhood. Those symptoms must be persistent and current. The accuracy of ADHD diagnosis in adults is important and, therefore, a diagnosis should only be made by a specialist who has specialized in the field of attention dysfunction. For a diagnosis to be accurate, the behavioral history of patients since childhood needs to be evaluated. In addition, interviews with patients' life partner, parents, family members or close associates will be required. Psychological tests and physical examinations can also be undertaken to establish whether one's condition is related to other conditions such as anxiety, learning disabilities, or affective disorders.

To diagnose ADHD in older teens and adults, they must have demonstrated the symptoms of different ADHD types in multiple settings. For instance, if an adult fails to hold down one job for a considerable period, a diagnosis could help unravel whether ADHD is the underlying cause behind this situation. Just like it is the case when diagnosing ADHD in kids, the symptoms must have been observed for a considerable period, and in different settings.

Adults who have struggled with ADHD unknowingly for years often have a sense of relief after a correct diagnosis of the disorder has been made. Typically, individuals who have unknowingly suffered from ADHD bring many negative perceptions about themselves into adulthood due to the effect that the condition has had on them. Once past and present behaviors that are related to ADHD have been brought into perspective, it is easy for one to face them head-on. This could perhaps explain why ADHD treatment in adults mostly entails psychotherapy since it helps them cope with whatever anger they might feel owing to the failure to diagnose the condition during their childhood or younger years.

Couples with ADHD

If an adult has ADHD, it is obvious that the first person who will be affected is his/her spouse/partner Needless to say, the disorder can put an end to even the closest of relationships. Symptoms such as procrastination, distraction, and impulsivity, can stir feelings such as hunger and frustration, besides hurting the other party's feelings. When such a situation occurs in both adults with ADHD and their partners can be affected and, consequently, drift apart. Nevertheless, the relationship can still thrive even one partner has ADHD. Proper treatment and coping tactics can help couples ward off the devastating effects of ADHD.

Couples' Expectation Guide on ADHD Marriage

Distraction

Distraction is among the commonest ADHD symptoms. If one of the couple has ADHD, chances are high that most times, he/she won't seem to listen whenever the other speaks to them. Such individuals may also constantly fail to follow through on any promises made to their partners. Love still exists, but they tend to get distracted by their phones, the TV, or, sometimes, just their own thoughts.

How to Deal With Distraction

The fact that one partner easily gets distracted, or tends to wander off whenever a discussion is being held, doesn't mean that he/she no longer cares about the other. Once this symptom is noticed over a prolonged period and in different settings, a diagnosis should be considered as soon as possible. Being open, in a calm manner, about feelings of how this makes the other feel is equally important. Bottling up feelings, anger, and emotion can lead to spousal resentment.

If the constant distraction is causing conversations to be a real problem, finding the most appropriate time when they get least distracted is a good idea. Sometimes, it helps to touch their arms when talking to them so that they notice the other's presence. This will make it hard for them to drift away. To connect with an ADHD partner during conversations, establish what makes them drift away. Thereafter, avoid situations that make them get distracted. In addition, keep conversations brief because it will be harder for them to become uninterested and distracted.

Hyper-focus

This is the opposite of distraction, and another symptom of ADHD. ADHD adults who experience hyperfocus tend to get so engrossed in an activity that it makes it hard to shift their attention away. Hyperfocus can be advantageous, especially in cases where it enhances an individual's productivity. Nonetheless, it can also be disastrous if left unchecked. Loved ones, in particular, are the ones who are likely to bear the brunt of hyperfocus because they might feel less important, simply because something that doesn't seem to be important has taken away their loved ones' attention.

Dealing With Hyperfocus

If a spouse is prone to spells of hyperfocus when undertaking certain activities, such as creating puzzles, it's best for the other to engage them elsewhere. Scheduling such activities far away from mealtimes or moments when partners need to interact with each other will help. Those who portray symptoms of hyperfocus can set alarms to track time that they spent on one activity. This will help them move to equally important activities when they realize that they are hyper-focused. Partners shouldn't take it personally if their spouses have the habit of being hyper-focused on other activities.

Forgetfulness

It's often the case that one partner thinks the other is being forgetful for the sake of it. The truth of the matter is that he/she could be battling with ADHD unknowingly. Without a diagnosis, a level of distrust could sink in towards the ADHD partner even with basic tasks. For the partner with ADHD and they don't realize this to be the case, they may end up feeling like a failure. Ultimately, anger will build up on both sides.

Forgetfulness Strategies

Forgetfulness isn't a character flaw like many people have been led to believe. If one partner has the tendency of forgetting even basic things, the other can make an effort to seek a diagnosis. Avoid labeling this ADHD symptom as being uncaring or being rude. Also, giving the ADHD partner lengthy lectures will only make him/her fall deeper into self-pity and resentment, towards the other. Focusing on working with your spouse to help him/her remember tasks that they are to undertake will help. A daily planner or task reminders on their phones will also come in handy.

Disorganization

ADHD adults are likely to have the disorganization trait. Such individuals are likely to leave their jobs unfinished or even skip their chores altogether, lose important documents, car keys, and phones. Disorganization not only leads to stress but also wastage. Trying to give a lecture to an adult with ADHD who is disorganized can leave him/her feeling controlled.

How to Cope With Disorganization

Whenever a spouse is disorganized, the other should try to sit him/her down and talk to them calmly. One maybe disorganized when undertaking some roles but can be more organized in others. Understanding each other's strengths when undertaking tasks will go a long way in preventing chore wars. Besides this, respecting the ADHD partner's habit of keeping items in certain spots might be difficult but will be rewarding. In as much that the placement of the items in those spots might look clumsy; it could be their way of keeping things organized.

Impulsivity

Adults who have the hyperactive form of ADHD tend to make impulsive decisions. They will act without thinking. In marriages, the main problem that hyperactive ADHD couples may experience is impulsive spending. One may have the habit of buying things out-of-the-blue without consulting the other, or considering the family unit's financial situation. Some of the items might even be irrelevant or might be viewed as being extravagant and inconsiderate. Either way, the underlying cause of the impulsivity could be ADHD. If a partner has risqué sexual habits, drives dangerously, or often blurts out unsuitable comments in social occasions, he/she could be driven by impulsivity.

Handling Impulsivity

Managing impulsivity in a marriage setting entails a lot of self-control, which can actually be learned. Aiding a partner to develop self-control in all situations can be done through role-playing, so that they learn how to act in different situations. If they have the habit of overspending on their credit cards, teaching them how to write shopping lists and also why they should leave their credit cards at home when going shopping will help. The most crucial thing about managing impulsivity is cutting out temptation. If the impulsive behaviors get out of hand, therapy definitely needs to be sought.

Procrastination

Everyone has a habit of putting off tasks that appear boring or difficult. In a marriage setting, this habit can be detrimental because relationships involve playing differing roles in the household and relationship. An ADHD adult who has the habit of procrastinating may not know how to undertake tasks, or they might feel overwhelmed. They only tend to get started when deadlines are on the horizon. This is a recipe for chaotic lifestyles, which may ultimately cause couples to drift apart.

Avoiding Procrastination

Most adults who tend to push forward their roles have the inattention type of ADHD. They feel overwhelmed by tasks that often appear too big to handle. Rather than letting them struggle with such tasks, the other partner can work with them to break the project into smaller tasks that are easy to tackle. Sharing duties within the task will give the other partner some company and support since it will make them tail off. ADHD adults shouldn't look at procrastination as a defect but rather as a trait that is manageable.

Mood Swings

Individuals who have ADHD often exhibit erratic behavior, which is characterized by a shift between spells of happiness and moodiness. They also have difficulty when it comes to controlling their emotions; they might want to lash out in anger when their moods set in simply because they feel anxious or frustrated. If this is the case and the ADHD us undiagnosed their behavior might compromise the relationship.

Managing Mood Swings

Normally, a partner's mood swings are caused by events happening around them. Therefore, lifestyle changes can go a long way in alleviating the erratic moods. A healthy diet, regular exercise, and ample sleep will go a long way in preventing the mood swings. Keep in mind that a spouse's moods swings can only be eased is he/she learns how to control their impulses. For the other partner, avoid topics and conversations that may lead to overreactions and flare-ups. In as much as their situation should be empathized with, an explanation as to their mood swings affect the other is important. With time, they will learn how to control their emotions.

ADHD And Intimacy

Couples who have ADHD often have problems as far as communication and intimacy are concerned. If you have ADHD, you may experience trouble paying attention to your partner. Your mind might wander even during the most intimate moments with your spouse. This will seem normal to you but nonetheless, your partner is likely to see it as lack of interest. With time, a lack of attention may breed resentment, which in turn causes spouses to drift apart. ADHD adults are also likely to be drawn to risky sexual behaviors such as unprotected sexual encounters. ADHD often lowers the level of neurotransmitters, thus putting you at risk of being impulsive and taking risks.

Married couples who have ADHD are bound to realize that the condition often affects their relationship in many ways. Distractibility and inattention, which are among the main ADHD symptoms, often subverts eroticism and romance. However, this doesn't mean that ADHD and intimacy cannot coexist. Couples should find a way of keeping their intimacy intact even when one of them has ADHD.

Spouses with ADHD must find a way of rebalancing their relationship. Similarly should work towards letting go of any resentment that might have cropped up as a result of the condition. Talking to a therapist can go a long way in helping rekindle the long-lost intimacy. ADHD couples who have kids should learn to share responsibilities pertaining to childcare, money and organization. Ultimately, their romance will be reawakened.

It is generally advisable for couples to address the big challenges that face their relationship while finding new ways of learning communication skills. This will not only bridge their differences but also minimize whatever resentment that might have cropped up. In this regard, couples need to hone their speaking and listening skills while discussing their challenges without being aggressive or listening defensively. This will help them maintain or discover their affection towards each other. When dealing with ADHD as a couple, it is always good to let the partner know how one feels.

ADHD at the Workplace

There are certain attributes that employers often look out for before hiring staff. These include excellent focus, speed, organization, an ability to meet deadlines, and attention to detail. If you have ADHD, meeting such requirements can be quite a challenge. Even when you are on the job, excelling in your roles ends up being a tall order, thus making it difficult for you to keep the job, let alone getting promoted. This shouldn't mean that you can't excel in a career if you have ADHD. Sometimes, the disorder can be an asset to you and your workmates.

How ADHD Affects Employment

Up to 9 million adults in the U.S. have ADHD. This represents a significant percentage of the American workforce. Studies have shown that adults with ADHD often struggle at work. A national survey indicated that only 50% of adults who have ADHD are able to maintain a full-time job. On the flipside, 72% of adults without ADHD can hold down a full-time job. Whenever ADHD adults land a job, they tend to earn slightly less than their colleagues who do not have the disorder.

The extent to which the disorder affects your employment outlook depends on its severity. While some individuals may only have problems when it comes to staying on one task, others find it hard to work all day without getting into a blow-up with their co-workers or superiors. Those who are severely affected by ADHD may end up moving from one job to another. In extreme cases, they even end up seeking disability benefits.

Generally, this behavioral disorder affects job performance in various ways. If you cannot sit still during meetings or you have difficulties staying focused and organized, it will be hard for you to stay on one job for a substantial amount of time. Typically, individuals battling with ADHD have trouble with working memory, attention, verbal fluency, and mental processing. These qualities are generally referred to as executive-function abilities, and they come in handy at the workplace. Within the work environment, it is easy for you to get depressed or have low self-esteem if you have difficulties completing your tasks within schedules or beating simple deadlines. This may make your situation even worse.

How ADHD Adults Can Succeed at Work

Adults who lack the ability to concentrate or are restless, often haven't been diagnosed with ADHD. If you experience any ADHD-related symptoms, it is advisable that you have the disorder diagnosed and managed accordingly. Once medication and therapy starts you will find it easier to manage your daily roles and even succeed in your career and social life. ADHD adults are often advised to work with career counselors when embarking on a job search. This goes a long way in helping them land jobs that match their abilities, needs, and interests. Depending on your ADHD, you may want to find employment in either a fast-paced environment, or a less rigid one.

Once you have landed a job, there are certain strategies that can help you manage your ADHD. Find peace in whatever work environment you find yourself in. Ask to be allocated a quiet working space where it won't be easy for you to get distracted. If you have trouble organizing your tasks and schedule, work with a colleague or superior who is well-organized so that you are guided through projects. Besides this, always maintain a daily planner with a to-do list and a calendar. Have electronic reminders about due dates and meetings to keep you updated with what you are supposed to do.

To keep your memory fresh, always take notes during meetings and also when making work-related phone calls. Add these notes to your diary and to-do lists. You should also schedule interruptions by setting aside specific periods for answering your calls or emails. This will ensure that your schedule and more important responsibilities are not interrupted. When undertaking tasks, you should set realistic goals for yourself while bearing in mind that you have ADHD. Break up every workday into a series of assignments and, thereafter, attempt to tackle each small assignment one at a time. In this regard, have a timer that will notify you when to move to the next task.

To effectively manage ADHD at work, it is advisable that you always reward yourself after completing tasks. Taking a break or even stepping out of the office for a break is a worthy reward. For bigger accomplishments, you should even consider buying yourself something that you've always wanted. To avoid a breakdown that typifies ADHD symptoms, you should be ready to delegate smaller tasks so that you can focus on more important ones. This will also prevent loss of focus as a result of distractions. What's more, you should always make it a habit to relax. This will help ramp up our energy levels, thus boosting your concentration.

How ADHD Can be Beneficial At Work

ADHD is categorized as a disability under the Americans with Disabilities Act. Employers are required to accommodate the needs of employees who have ADHD without discriminating against them. You need to be bold enough to inform your employer that you have ADHD. Unbeknown to many people, ADHD can be used to a positive effect at work. The impulsiveness, desire to try out new things, and restlessness can be great assets if harnessed properly. These ADHD symptoms particularly come in handy if you run your own business. The trick lies in finding a career that suits you and uses your boundless energy, creativity, and other strengths to your benefit.

With necessary support, adults who have ADHD can be productive members of the workplace. For instance, an ADHD symptom such as hyperfocus ought to be harnessed so that these individuals are allowed to work on projects that they are most interested in. They are likely to focus intensely on such projects, something that will ultimately result in positive results.

Hyperfocus is advantageous owing to the fact that it can help employees to channel their attention and energy into whatever projects that they handle. The ability to focus for hours on end particularly comes in handy in careers such as science, writing, and art. ADHD adults are generally advised not to wallow in their condition. Instead, they should be proud of the out-of-the-box thinking, passion, and drive that it brings. Looking at the condition in a positive light will go a long way in helping them manage it.

The lack of awareness about ADHD means that many adult patients end up being misunderstood or misinterpreted at their workplaces due to their inconsistency. As a result, many of them struggle to hold down one job for a considerable period. Proper diagnosis and management of the condition can go a long way in enabling ADHD adults to make the most of their talents.

Chapter 4: Medical and Treatment Guidance for ADHD

Medication for ADHD Types

The three types of ADHD exhibit varying symptoms and, as a result, they should be treated differently. Besides differences in medications used, the kind of therapy that ought to be offered for the three ADHD types also varies. In addition, treatment for kids with ADHD varies from treatment offered to adults.

Medication for Hypersensitive-Impulsive ADHD Type

Individuals who have this type of ADHD often exhibit strong emotional reaction towards things and circumstances that "normal" people take in their stride. The heightened and over-the-top reactions are typically emotional in nature, and may arise from rather negative or positive situations. It isn't unusual for individuals who have hypersensitive-impulsive ADHD to be physically sensitive to common senses such as light, sound, and touch. More than 50% of individuals with this ADHD type have difficulties with emotional regulation and, therefore, they experience symptoms such as temper outbursts, impulsivity, mood fluctuations, and low tolerance levels.

Antidepressants are the most widely-used medicines as far as the treatment of hypersensitive-impulsive ADHD is concerned. Common antidepressants used to treat this disorder include bupropion, desipramine, imipramine, and nortriptyline. Each of these medicines has its side effects, but the severity of the symptoms depends on the dosage with which the medicines are administered. Bupropion may cause headaches in rare cases. It also increases the risk of seizures and, therefore, an individual's medical history ought to be evaluated before the drug is administered. Desipramine isn't recommended for use among children with hypersensitive-impulsive ADHD. The drug is associated with some rare cases of heart ailments. Imipramine may cause several side effects, including fatigue, anxiety, stomach upsets, increased risk of arrhythmias, elevated heartbeat, and dry mouth. These side effects may also be present in individuals with hypersensitive-impulsive ADHD who are treated with nortriptyline.

Generally, antidepressants are considered to be safe, especially if the dosage is administered by a professional. Rarely do serious problems arise after the drugs have been administered. Besides this, not all hypersensitive-impulsive patients will exhibit the aforementioned side effects once these drugs have been administered.

Medication for Inattentive ADHD

Individuals suffering from inattentive ADHD often have problems staying alert over longer periods. In most cases, stimulant medication is recommended to enable their brains to send and receive signals, thus enabling them to pay attention for longer periods, and also to think more clearly. The most common medications used to manage inattentive ADHD include amphetamine-based and methylphenidate-based medicines. Once inattentive ADHD has been diagnosed, the medical practitioner will recommend a low dose of the aforementioned medicines to see whether your symptoms will be controlled. If it doesn't, the dose may be slowly increased.

Most medicines used to treat inattentive ADHD come in short-term and long-term acting forms. The former typically wear off in around 4 hours. Therefore, you are required to take them once or twice daily. On the other hand, long-acting stimulants wear off after 8-12 hours. You are only required to take these once a day. For inattentive ADHD treatment, to achieve the most suitable outcome, it is advisable that you talk with your doctor so that you decide on the medication that works best for you. In this regard, you should consider your daily routine so that you figure out the best schedule for taking your medication.

ADHD patients should avoid taking stimulants if they have serious health disorders such as glaucoma, a history of substance and alcohol abuse, and heart disease. If you are taking an antidepressant while under treatment for inattentive ADHD, you should consult your doctor before embarking on stimulant medication. You also need to keep in mind that stimulants cause side effects, such as mouth dryness, headaches, insomnia, and loss of appetite. If you also take medication via patches on your skin, the skin color in those specific areas is likely to change. You shouldn't be worried about the side effects of stimulant medication because, in most cases, they disappear on their own within a few days or weeks of commencing medication. If you feel that the side effects are a bother, consult your doctor so that a different drug is prescribed to you, or the dosage is changed.

Non-Stimulant Medication for ADHD

Non-stimulant medication can also be used to treat ADHD. This route is normally taken when treating combined type ADHD. In addition, non-stimulant medication can be used on individuals who experience drastic side effects to stimulant medication. Anti-stimulants, such as atomoxetine are administered to raise chemical levels in the brains of ADHD patients, helping to control their behavior. These usually take several weeks to start working and if they are administered to you, you may experience side effects such as heartburn, constipation, and diminished sex drive; all of which will wear off in time. In case you cannot take other ADHD medication, your doctor may prescribe either clonidine or guanfacine, which are blood pressure drugs that can help you manage ADHD symptoms such as hyperactivity and impulsivity.

Treatment in Kids

To treat ADHD among kids effectively, families need to work with the healthcare professional who diagnosed the disorder in the first place. According to the Multimodal Treatment Study of Children with Attention Deficit Hyperactivity Disorder (MTA), one intervention cannot work in isolation as far as the treatment of ADHD is concerned. Medical management ought to be blended with behavioral treatment and routine community care for optimal outcomes to be attained.

Most kids who are diagnosed with this behavioral disorder are given medication. Stimulants and methylphenidates are the most common medications used. It is always advisable that children only be introduced to medication after behavioral therapy has been undertaken. Keep in mind that, when it comes to ADHD, no individual treatment strategy works for every child. Besides this, children sometimes have adverse side effects when subjected to a particular medication. In such situations, that particular treatment will be rendered unacceptable.

Medical Interventions for ADHD Kids

For years, various medicines have been used in the treatment of ADHD among kids. Generally, these medications only treat symptoms of the disorder. Stimulants have for long been regarded as the most effective medication as far as managing the symptoms of ADHD is concerned. Stimulants are often used to lower kids' impulsivity and hyperactivity thus improving their ability to focus on one activity at a time. This allows them to work and even learn new skills. Amphetamines are approved for use on ADHD children who are between the ages of 3 and 5. On the other hand, methylphenidates are typically used to treat the symptoms of ADHD among kids who are older than. Some of the amphetamines that are prescribed for kids with ADHD are meant to improve their physical coordination. The prescribing physician and the diagnosing specialist ought to work together to determine the right medication and dosage for each individual case.

Stimulants that are used to remedy ADHD among children are generally considered to be quite safe since they do not make the kids feel "high." Nevertheless, some kids may still feel funny or slightly different after using this medication. Stimulants used to treat ADHD among kids do not lead to dependence or drug abuse.

A paltry percentage of kids with ADHD are not helped by stimulant medication. Other medications can also be prescribed if ADHD occurs alongside another disorder. This includes antidepressants, which are typically administered to reduce anxiety or depression.

When using medicines as part of the interventions against ADHD symptoms, it is important to take note of a number of facts. Medications improve kids' focus thus helping them improve in school and in their overall social interactions. In addition, more than 80% of kids who need medication to mitigate the symptoms of ADHD will still need it when they enter their teenage years. 50% of them will need medication as adults.

Medication and behavioral therapy go a long way in mitigating ADHD among kids. Nevertheless, family members play the most crucial part. For this reason, both ADHD kids and their family members need special help since it will help them develop strategies for managing behavior patterns. Mental health professionals may be needed to counsel both the kids and their families in view of helping them develop new attitudes, skills, and ways of relating with each other. When counseling children who have ADHD, therapists should help them learn ways of feeling better about themselves. They should also help the kids identify and work on their strengths besides learning how to cope with problems that they face in their lives. In addition, they should also be taught how to manage their attention and aggression.

Every member of the family will be affected if a child has ADHD. Consequently, the entire family will need help so that everyone learns how to cope with the condition. Since kids with ADHD often have disruptive behaviors, therapists should focus on finding ways of handling such behaviors. This may entail teaching parents and other family members some techniques for coping with the behaviors and how to improve them.

Psychotherapy doesn't address the underlying causes or symptoms of ADHD. It basically entails the kids and their families talking to the therapist about upsetting feelings and thoughts. This helps them explore self-defeating behavioral patterns besides learning alternative ways of handling their emotions. As family members and parents talk to therapists, they will be able to understand how to deal with the disorder in a better way.

Behavioral therapists help ADHD kids and their families to develop ways of handling immediate issues that may arise. Rather than helping the kids understand their feelings and actions, behavioral therapy helps them change their thinking and, consequently, leads to changes in their behavior. This kind of support is akin to practical assistance, which helps them become more organized when undertaking their tasks, as well as helping them deal with emotionally-charged events.

Social-skills training can help children who have ADHD to learn new behaviors. This basically involves therapists discussing with the kids and their families appropriate behaviors that help build and maintain social relationships, such as waiting for a turn, responding to teasing, and asking for help. For instance, the kids might be taught how to read people's facial expressions and voice tones, so that they learn how to respond appropriately.

Support groups can be used to help parents connect with other parents whose kids are suffering from ADHD. Support groups members can meet on a regular basis and listen to behavioral experts so that they learn how best to deal with their kids' situation. Support groups similarly enable parents to share their successes and failures as far as managing their ADHD is concerned. They can also obtain referrals to experts and pertinent information in dealing with ADHD.

Parental skills training is offered either in special classes or by behavioral therapists to parents, with the objective of giving them techniques for managing their kids' behavior. The most common technique is rewarding good behavior and isolating them when they misbehave. This system of rewards and sanctions is an effective way of modifying a kid's behavior.

When kids are rewarded for good behavior or completing tasks, they identify desirable behaviors that they should uphold, and undesirable behaviors to avoid. Over time, such techniques help ADHD kids to learn how to control their behavior and thus choose those ones that are desirable. When handling their ADHD kids, parents also need to learn ways of structuring situations in a manner that allows their kids to succeed. This includes allowing them to interact with several playmates at a time. Their children won't be overstimulated to be hyperactive or impulsive, or inattentive in such cases. If your kid has difficulties completing tasks, you can help them learn to do so by dividing large tasks into smaller bits. The kid should be praised and rewarded as he/she completes the smaller tasks. Parents should also learn how to use stress management techniques such as relaxation methods, exercise, and meditation. This will increase their tolerance for frustration thus enabling them to respond more calmly to their kid's behavior.

Strategies for Family with ADHD

Medication and behavioral therapy go a long way in mitigating ADHD among kids. Nevertheless, family members play the most crucial part. For this reason, both ADHD kids and their family members need special help, for it will help them develop strategies for managing behavior patterns. Mental health professionals may be needed to counsel both the kids and their families in view of helping them develop new attitudes, skills, and ways of relating with each other. When counseling children who have ADHD, therapists should help them learn ways of feeling better about themselves. They should also help the kids identify and work on their strengths besides learning how to cope with problems that they face in their lives. In addition, they should also be taught how to manage their attention and aggression.

Every member of the family is most likely to be affected if one of your kids has ADHD. Consequently, the entire family will need help so that everyone learns how to cope with the condition. Since kids with ADHD often have disruptive behaviors, therapists should focus on finding ways of handling such behaviors. This may entail teaching parents and other family members some techniques for coping with the behaviors and how to improve them.

Psychotherapy doesn't address the underlying causes or symptoms of ADHD. It basically entails the kids and their families talking to the therapist about upsetting feelings and thoughts. This helps them explore self-defeating behavioral patterns besides learning alternative ways of handling their emotions. As family members and parents talk to therapists, they will be able to understand how to deal with the disorder in a better way.

Behavioral therapists help ADHD kids and their families to develop ways of handling immediate issues that may arise. Rather than helping the kids understand their feelings and actions, behavioral therapy helps them change their thinking and, consequently, leads to changes in their behavior. This kind of support to the kids and their family members is akin to practical assistance, which helps them become more organized when undertaking their tasks, besides helping them deal with emotionally-charged events.

On the other hand, social skills training helps children who have ADHD to learn new behaviors. This basically involves therapists discussing with the kids and their families appropriate behaviors that help build and maintain social relationships, such as waiting for a turn, responding to teasing, and asking for help. For instance, the kids might be taught how to read people's facial expressions and voice tones so that they learn how to respond appropriately. Social skills training help family members and the kids themselves develop ways of socializing.

Support groups can be used to help parents connect with other parents whose kids are suffering from ADHD. Support groups members can meet on a regular basis and listen to behavioral experts so that they learn how best to deal with their kids' situation. They also enable parents to share their successes and failures as far as managing ADHD and are a great place to obtain referrals to experts and pertinent information in dealing with ADHD.

Parental skills training is offered either in special classes or behavioral therapists to parents with the objective of giving them techniques for managing their kids' behavior. The most common technique is rewarding good behavior and isolating them when they misbehave. When kids are rewarded for good behavior or completing tasks, they identify desirable behaviors that they should uphold, and undesirable behaviors to avoid. Over time, such techniques help ADHD kids to learn how to control their behavior and thus choose those ones that are desirable.

When handling their ADHD kids, parents also need to learn ways of structuring situations in a manner that allows their kids to succeed. This includes allowing them to interact with several playmates at a time, avoiding overstimulation and situations that will cause them to be hyperactive or impulsive. If your kid has difficulties completing tasks, you can help them learn to do so by dividing large tasks into smaller bits. They should be praised and rewarded as he/she completes the smaller tasks.

Parents should also learn how to use stress management techniques, such as relaxation methods, exercise, and meditation. This will increase their tolerance for frustration, thus enabling them to respond more calmly to their child's behavior.

Home Activities and Simple Exercises for Child with ADHD

Generally, children with ADHD need help to organize their daily activities. In this regard, there are some simple exercises and home activities that come in handy. Treating ADHD starts with scheduling their activities in such a way that they have a similar routine on a daily basis. Spontaneous behavior can be averted if ADHD kids are tuned to adhere to the same routine from the time they wake up until they go to bed. The schedule ought to incorporate activities such as homework time, outdoor recreation, and indoor activities, and should be put somewhere they can easily see to ensure memorization. In case there is any change in the schedule, ensure that the change is communicated to your kids in advance.

Parents and family members should also organize items needed on a daily basis. This will go a long way in preventing spontaneous and unpredictable reactions, which are likely to manifest when ADHD kids fail to find whatever they are looking for. In this regard, you should consider setting aside a place for everything. Besides this, ensure that everything is kept in its place, including school supplies, clothing, and backpacks.

You should also consider using notebook and homework reminders to keep your kids apprised of what he/she should be doing at a particular time. This comes in handy when they are doing school-related chores such as assignments. In line with this, stress to them why it is important to write down all assignments that they are given at school and coming home with the needed books. This way, it will be difficult for them to forget about their assignments. You should take note of the fact that ADHD children need consistent rules that are easy to understand and abide by. If the rules that you lay down for them are followed, ensure that you give appropriate rewards. Always look out for any good behavior that they exhibit and praise it accordingly.

Managing ADHD within the School Environment

The fact that you have a child with ADHD doesn't mean that he/she shouldn't be given an opportunity to attend school. Actually, the social interactions that ADHD kids have at a school, play a significant role as far as behavioral change is concerned. ADHD isn't only managed within the home environment but also at school. Even though you won't be at school with your kid, there are certain measures that you can take to ensure that the disorder is managed within their learning environment.

When it comes to the management of ADHD within the school environment, you should keep in mind the fact that you are your kid's best advocate. To effectively play this role, you need to be as conversant as possible with this behavioral disorder. Learn everything you can about ADHD and the effect that it has on your kid's behavior within the home environment, at school, and in diverse social situations. If your kid has portrayed ADHD symptoms since early on in his/her life, and the disorder has been diagnosed and treated using a combination of behavioral therapy and medical interventions, you should let teachers know about it. This will put them in a position to understand your kid's behavior. Likewise, they will know how best to handle that kid in the new setting, away from the home environment.

In case your child has entered the school system and is having problems that lead you to suspect that he/she has ADHD, it is advisable that you either seek advice from a behavioral expert. Besides this, you can have an evaluation undertaken by the local school district. Generally, schools are mandated to evaluate kids who they suspect to have behavioral disabilities, including ADHD. This is more so the case if the disorder is affecting their academic work and social interactions with teachers and fellow learners. If you think that your school-going ADHD child isn't learning as he/she should make it a point to establish who you need to contact within the school system. Thereafter, you can request that the school undertake an evaluation.

For many years, many schools were reluctant to admit children with ADHD, or even evaluate those already within the system who are suspected of having the disorder. Nevertheless, laws have been made making it mandatory for schools to evaluate kids, in a bid to establish whether their poor academic performance or social skills are caused by behavioral disorders such as ADHD. Once your kid is diagnosed with ADHD, it is obvious that he/she qualifies for specialized educational services. In line with this, the child's school must work with you to assess his/her strengths and weaknesses in view of coming up with an individualized educational program. With such a program in place, it will be easy to gauge the kid's performance even when he/she transitions to a different school.

ADHD and Teenage Transition

As your kid grows older and transitions into a teenager, ADHD stays with him/her. By this time, you should have learned how to manage the symptoms of the disorder as your child proceeds to middle school and, thereafter, junior high. In as much as the child may have been evaluated periodically through the years, it is good practice to undertake another re-evaluation as teenage years set in. Generally, the teenage years are challenging for many children, regardless of whether they have a behavioral disorder or not. Children with ADHD, in particular, find their teenage years even more stressful because, in addition to their condition, they have to battle with typical adolescent problems such as peer pressure, fear of failure in school and socially, and low self-esteem. These, among other challenges, make it hard for ADHD children to cope with adolescence compared to "normal" teens.

Like every teenager, ADHD teens experience the desire to be independent and try new or forbidden things, such as sexual activity, drugs, and alcohol. Needless to say, engaging in such behaviors often leads to undesirable consequences. Owing to the numerous challenges that ADHD teens face, it is advisable that clear rules be laid down and adhered to. Rules meant to guide the behavior of ADHD teens should not only be straightforward but also easy to understand. There also needs to be seamless communication between parents and their teens because, unlike during their younger years, teens can easily express themselves. Therefore, parents should let them understand the reasons behind each rule. These rules should stipulate how teens should behave, both at home and outside the home environment.

Since ADHD adolescents are emotionally fragile, parents ought to respond calmly whenever they break rules. Punishment should be used sparingly and, just like as it is the case with pre-school children, time-outs should be used to control inappropriate behavior. Typically, hot temper and impulsivity accompany ADHD amongst teenagers. Therefore, time alone can help them calm down and return to their senses.

As ADHD teenagers increasingly spend more time away from the home environment, there will be demands such as the use of family cars and later curfews. When such requests are made, listen to them carefully and give concise reasons for your opinions. Learn to negotiate and compromise since this will ultimately prove helpful.

Treatment of ADHD in Adults

Therapy

The idea of ADHD therapy for adults is to help them know how best they can manage their condition. It similarly helps them learn how to change whatever long-standing poor self-image that they might have. They do so by examining their experiences with the disorder in years gone by, and how to avoid the not-so-good ones.

Psychotherapy is often used alongside medical interventions to manage ADHD and its symptoms in adults. You have to keep in mind the fact that even though medication alleviates some of the symptoms of ADHD, individuals ought to make a deliberate effort to sign up for both individual therapy and psycho-education sessions. Psychotherapy for adults' ADHD classes typically entails teaching patients how to embrace their condition without feeling bitter about the impact that it might have had on their lives.

Those who are forgetful can use props and reminders to keep them apprised of their schedules. Likewise, ADHD adults who find it cumbersome to complete tasks can have those tasks broken down into smaller portions. The completion of individual mini-tasks will give them a sense of accomplishment. What's more, it is advisable that adult ADHD individuals learn as much as they can about the disorder since it will put them in a good position to face it.

The success of psychotherapy sessions for ADHD adults starts with them remembering minor routines; keeping the appointment time with the therapist is a good start. This is a step in the right direction and will help them learn how to keep subsequent appointments with the therapists and any other people that they are to meet in future.

In most cases, therapists encourage ADHD adults who are seeking treatment to adjust to whatever changes that the therapy sessions might have brought to their lives. Such changes may include the apparent loss of impulsivity, a diminished love for risk-taking, and the new sense of thinking before making any decisions. Such changes are likely to be worrisome to some patients and, therefore, the therapist needs to explain this to them once they start experiencing the changes. As adult ADHD patients begin experiencing minor success in their ability to organize what would hitherto be complex situations, it becomes easy for them to appreciate and embrace ADHD characteristics that are positive. These include boundless warmth, energy, and enthusiasm.

Risks of Untreated Adult ADHD

Like has been mentioned earlier, ADHD in adults often remains undetected in most cases. Untreated ADHD among both kids and adults tends to lead to a myriad of problems throughout one's life. Due to the impulsiveness and short attention spans that characterize individuals with ADHD, leaving the condition unattended makes it hard for them to succeed in school, climb the career ladder, and build strong relationships. Simply put, the disorder affects all aspects of an individual's life if it is left untreated.

Adults who have ADHD that is undetected and untreated often find it difficult to manage their emotions and ensuing reactions. As a result, they end up experiencing social problems, since they may not know how best to take turns, interact with others, or even react appropriately in certain situations. Without treatment and therapy, their social circle may be limited to close family members' due to a lack of the ability to make and keep friends. Many people unknowingly regard ADHD adults as being hard to deal with. In the end, they shun them, something that often leads such individuals to suffer from depression and a lack of self-esteem.

Adults who have untreated ADHD are also more likely to get into car accidents, be in trouble with the law, or have gambling problems due to impulsivity. Research indicates that up to 40% of prison inmates have a form of ADHD. In most of these cases, the disorder is either undiagnosed or untreated. This clearly suggests that had these individuals been diagnosed and treated for ADHD early enough, actions that led to their incarceration may not have occurred in the first place.

How Long Should ADHD Medication be Administered?

The amount of time that ADHD medication is administered generally depends on the severity of the disorder and the potency of the drug being used. In children, teens, and college students, it is recommended that ADHD medication is administered throughout their school year so that they can concentrate better in class.

Beyond college, the length of treatment will depend on an individual's situation and the level of general pressure from external factors such as work, home, or in social situations, and how they are handling them. Whether one stays on medication at all times is a personal decision. You have to keep in mind that assists ADHD patients maintain whatever positive improvements they may have made in their lives. This way, it will be possible for them to keep making positive and meaningful changes going forward.

Most patients who seek treatment for ADHD often seek interventions for disorders that go beyond ADHD. This is why it is advisable to combine medication and therapy, or any other non-pharmacological interventions that a medical practitioner may deem fit. In most cases, the baggage that accompanies ADHD is usually part of the problem and, therefore, doctors must also focus on the. A significant number of emotional issues that most ADHD patients experience have something to do with them feeling bad about themselves and that they feel incapable of being competent. The situation is compounded by the fact that before ADHD gets diagnosed, many patients receive negative feedback from their friends, colleagues, and family members who typically consider them to be lazy and not good enough.

Should Patients Consider Psychotherapy?

Talking therapy and cognitive-behavioral therapy should be part and parcel of ADHD treatment. This intervention is particularly recommended to adults who have ADHD since it will help them hone their organizational skills. If someone has a history of other mental issues, they should consider talking therapy. If ADHD is the primary behavioral disorder, the doctor will probably focus on enhancing executive functions, which include organizational skills, time management, and planning.

Therapy for ADHD also involves helping patients to gain more mastery over their emotions and reactions. Behavioral therapy with specific goals can address the symptoms and behaviors that are deemed to be detrimental and problematic. For instance, patients who have difficulties keeping to appointments certainly have problems with planning their time. To remedy this, the therapist will try finding ways through which that patient can learn how to maintain a calendar. The success of therapy is hinged on the ability of the practitioner to help patients make changes in their lives, unlearn bad habits, plan better, react to situations in a more appropriate manner, and listen better.

ADHD Coaching

In recent years, there has been the emergence of ADHD coaching. This intervention not only offers specific problem-solving but also works effectively for severe cases. ADHD is akin to situations where there is a learner and a tutor, and involves working on specific issues that a patient might be experiencing. Pairing ADHD patients with coaches for sessions of up to 8 weeks improves their organizational ability, besides reducing anger levels that most of them might have maintained for up to a year.

Generally, ADHD coaching targets specific areas of weaknesses, including low motivation, poor organizational skills, impulsivity, poor anger control, and attention problems. When these specific problems are addressed, it is easy to put patients back on track. Most coaches who offer ADHD coaching are not therapists or medical experts. Personal coaching helps patients to understand both the nature of ADHD and the impact that the condition had in their lives. Similarly, it helps patients learn ways of facing obstacles and focus on their goals. Coaches work with patients to create strategies, structures, and build skills that help them address ADHD-related issues such as organization, self-esteem, and time management. Therefore, you should only choose one who has a history of working with ADHD patients.

Can ADHD Be Treated Without Drugs?

The short answer to this is, "yes." Once a positive ADHD diagnosis has been made, the long trek through the pharmaceutical world begins. Medication is the preferred intervention for ADHD since it is effective for up to 80% of patients. When ADHD is diagnosed, many people start worrying about the medication side effects. On paper, these look scary and, therefore, patients and their family members often prefer exhausting other ADHD treatment before medication is considered.

In children, it is recommended that medication only starts after they start going to school. Before that, behavioral therapy should be used instead of drugs. Quite often, patients inquire whether they can try out other treatments before they consider medicine. When mitigating the symptoms of ADHD in kids, it is always advisable for parents to find out about other treatments that work for their kids before they turn to medication. Behavioral therapy alone can be effective, especially in pre-school kids who are only showing unfocused and inattentive symptoms. In older kids and adults, a combination of medicine and behavioral treatment works best.

Alternative Interventions to Medicines and Therapy

Apart from medicine and therapy, there are other interventions that can help to manage symptoms of ADHD, and for the individual to live a "normal" life. For instance, getting enough sleep can be beneficial to kids with ADHD since it particularly helps with impulsivity and restlessness.

Sleep

Most kids who have ADHD also suffer from sleep disorders. In such cases, the presence of each disorder makes the other even worse. The most common sleep disorder for children with ADHD is the inability to settle down, preventing them from falling asleep. They end up experiencing exhaustion the following day, something that makes them even more restless. While some medical practitioners recommend the use of sleeping aids, such as melatonin, parents should start with practicing good sleep habits. This includes having consistent bedtime routines even on weekends, keeping kids' bedrooms dark, and creating a calming winding-down ritual every night.

Exercise

Plenty of exercise can also help both ADHD adults and children to manage their symptoms more effectively. In this regard, there's a need for patients to have plenty of opportunities for exercising at appropriate times. Research indicates that up to 30 minutes of exercise helps kids who have ADHD to be more focused and organized in their activities. Water has a natural calming effect, and so swimming can be a very popular form of exercise for people with ADHD thus having a knock-on calming effect to other areas of their lives.

Exercise isn't only good for keeping the body fit. It also helps maintain brain health. Whenever you exercise, the brain releases neurotransmitters such as dopamine, which enhances clear thinking and attention. Individuals who have ADHD often tend to have low levels of dopamine in their brains. Exercising helps ease anxiety and stress, both in ADHD kids and adults. It also improves impulse control, thus reducing compulsive behavior.

Those with ADHD who regularly exercise also have improved working memory and enhanced executive function. This enables them to plan and organize their activities more effectively, besides remembering specific details. Exercising also increases the level of the brain-derived neurotropic factor, a protein that enhances memory and learning, and is usually in short supply among individuals who are suffering from ADHD.

Meditation and Mindfulness

Recent studies have unraveled that mindfulness and meditation can help individuals with ADHD cope better with the disorder. Mindfulness and meditation typically involve learning how to become more aware, sharpen focus, and practice self-control through breathing. When those with ADHD complete a mindfulness training program, they are likely to exhibit fewer symptoms of the disorder. Meditation can also control impulsivity because patients learn to control their thoughts before doing anything.

Meditation can go a long way in counteracting the stress of an adrenaline rush. When the word "meditation" is mentioned, many people who have ADHD may think that it can never apply to them. Meditation is among the most effective self-help techniques that can help people with ADHD stay calm. Meditation generally involves observing your moment-to-moment feelings and thoughts, with the objective of calming your mind and improving your focus. Unlike other treatments used to manage the symptoms of ADHD, meditation doesn't require any prescription, nor those seemingly endless trips to a therapist's office; you can meditate from the comfort of your bedroom.

Just the same way that we exercise to strengthen a specific part of our bodies, mindful meditation seeks to strengthen your ability to manage your reactions. It, similarly, helps you control your attention. If done correctly, it will help you learn ways of observing yourself and focus on a desired result. Mindful meditation itself is quite easy and doesn't require the presence of a guru.

Contrary to information that has been peddled in the public domain, meditation is easy, and you can't fail at it. You only need to get comfortable, find your comfort zone, and tone down from your full, high-speed adrenaline mode. Meditation trains you to control your wandering mind and bring it back to the moment before you become distracted. What's more, it makes you aware of your emotions, thus making you less vulnerable to impulsive behavior. It also raises the level of dopamine in your body, which is usually in short supply in individuals who have ADHD. Simply put, mindful meditation is an impulse control strategy.

Apart from mindful meditation, yoga can also be used to manage the often destructive symptoms of hyperactive-impulsive ADHD. It also increased dopamine levels in the brain, as well as strengthening the prefrontal cortex. A study among ADHD kids and adults established that those who practice yoga 20 minutes twice weekly for eight weeks made a significant improvement in their focus and attention, something that put them a better position to handle their condition. The use of mindful meditation and yoga to manage the symptoms of ADHD may look like an unexpected match but nonetheless, it significantly improves brain executive functions such as attention, concentration, and memory.

Recommended Food & Supplements to help with ADHD

Apart from medicine, therapy, and exercise, there are a number of foods and supplements that can help ADHD patients fight off detrimental symptoms. Some of the so-called alternative treatments for ADHD are inexpensive, easy to administer, and relatively safe, without side effects. However, the indicating that work faces strong arguments that this isn't the case. It is just the same with existing claims that sugar causes ADHD. Much controversy surrounding the link between sugar and ADHD still exists. The main question is whether or not sugar leads to hyperactivity. In as much as there is no proof to show that sugar leads to hyperactivity, many people still wonder why individuals seem to become hyperactive when they consume sugar in significant quantities.

Supplements Used to Manage ADHD Symptoms

1. Zinc
Some studies have suggested that kids who have ADHD have low zinc levels in their bodies. Zinc, which helps to enhance brain health, is one of the most essential minerals. Zinc deficiency not only affects other nutrients but also impacts on the brain function. Incorporating zinc-based supplements alleviates the symptoms of impulsivity, hyperactivity, and social problems, which characterize those with ADHD. Therefore, it can be said that taking zinc supplements can go a long way in improving some of the symptoms that ADHD individuals exhibit. Foods that are rich in zinc include seafood, poultry, red meat, beans, nuts, dairy products, fortified cereals, and whole grains.

2. Omega-3 Fatty Acids
There is proof that eating a diet rich in omega-3 fatty acids can improve ADHD symptoms. This supplement can be found in fish oil, and helps enhance the mental coordination of those with ADHD especially kids. They also ought to improve the ability to organize and plan. Vayarin, an FDA-approved supplement, is the most common and widely-used omega-3 fatty acid used by those with ADHD.

3. Iron
Some studies have attempted to link ADHD with low iron levels. One such study has proved that iron deficiency increases

the risk of mental disorders among kids and young adults. Iron is essential in the production of dopamine and norepinephrine, which are neurotransmitters that regulate emotions, stress, and the brain's reward system. According to medical practitioners, iron supplements can help relieve the symptoms of ADHD, especially in people who have an iron deficiency. It's important that there's an awareness surrounding the toxicity of over consuming iron. Therefore, a doctor should be consulted prior to taking iron supplements.

4. Magnesium

This is an important mineral that contributes significantly to brain health. Magnesium deficiency causes mental confusion, shortened attention span, and irritability however; you might not notice the benefits of supplementation if you're not magnesium deficient. Just like the case with iron, it is important to consult a doctor before you embark on the use of magnesium. When used in high doses, this supplement can lead to diarrhea, cramps, and nausea.

Herbs for ADHD

In recent years, there has been a growing popularity for the use of herbal remedies to manage ADHD symptoms. Just because herbal remedies are natural, it doesn't automatically mean that they are effective when compared to traditional treatments.

The following are some of the herbal remedies used to treat ADHD.

1. Korean Ginseng

An observational study meant to establish the effectiveness of Korean ginseng on children with ADHD established that the herb significantly reduces hyperactive behavior.

2. Valerian Root

It has been found that this herb can significantly increase concentration in ADHD individuals by up to 50% while decreasing hyperactivity. It also decreases impulsiveness while improving social behavior and sleep. These findings make it an effective treatment alongside other interventions.

ADHD Diets

There is no scientific proof that ADHD is caused by nutritional or diet problems. Nevertheless, research indicates that some foods may play a role in worsening or improving the symptoms of ADHD. Your eating habits go a long way in helping the brain function better. This, in turn, lessens typical ADHD symptoms such as a lack of focus and restlessness.

Generally, the main assumption that exists as far as the ADHD diet is concerned is that some of the foods that we eat either make ADHD symptoms better or worse. Elimination diets have also become popular. This mainly entails avoiding foods or ingredients that might trigger certain ADHD-related behaviors, thus worsening symptoms. For example, some flavorings, colorings, and preservatives increase hyperactivity among kids. The American Academy of Pediatrics states that eliminating some food colorings and preservatives can go a long way in mitigating some symptoms of hyperactive-impulsive ADHD.

The main consensus that exists when it comes to ADHD diets is that any food that is good for the brain improves the symptoms of ADHD. Therefore, you should consider eating high-protein diets comprising items such as beans, meat, cheese, and nuts, since they improve concentration, aside from helping certain medicine to work better.

It is also advisable to consume fewer simple carbohydrates such as candy, corn, and sugar since they are thought to increase hyperactivity. On the flipside, it is advisable to increase the intake of complex carbohydrates such as oranges, pears, tangerines, apples, grapefruit, and kiwi since they improve sleep, as well as reducing anxiety.

Chapter 5: ADHD and Other Mental Disorders

ADHD With Learning Disabilities in a Child

Many parents have been mistakenly led to believe that ADHD is a type of learning disability. This could be perhaps attributed to the fact that generally, the two disorders occur concurrently. Up to 30% of kids who have ADHD have a form of a learning disorder. According to child psychiatrists, having either of the conditions makes the other likely to occur, too. Thus, it goes without saying that ADHD can lead to learning difficulties in children. This is attested the fact that typically, ADHD children find it hard to focus in class and other activities for long enough. They similarly have trouble following instructions and directions. This doesn't however, mean that ADHD is a learning disability.

The distinctions between ADHD and learning difficulties have been shifting. In as much as the two disorders largely overlap, each has its own diagnostic criteria. Generally, there are several learning disabilities, and a child may have more than one of these. When either a parent or teacher suspects that a child has a learning disability, a psycho-educational test must be immediately conducted to confirm it. This test basically evaluates kids' intelligence or ability versus their achievement on standardized tests. Children who have learning disabilities often have average or above average IQ, however, often encounter difficulties when it comes to the processing and retrieval of information. This explains why they don't perform well in school tests.

Just like learning difficulties, ADHD also affects kids' ability to learn. Children who have ADHD have a number of brain function impairments, which makes them hyperactive, inattentive, or impulsive. As a result, these kids may seem to have learning difficulties simply because they are often hampered from acquiring working skills and information due to either their hyperactive behavior or inattentiveness.

What Are Some of the Most Common Learning Disabilities?

The most prevalent learning disabilities, which often get confused with ADHD, are:

- **Dyslexia.** This language disability mainly hinders kids' ability to understand and process written words. In some cases, dyslexia is referred to as a reading disability/disorder.

- **Dyscalculia.** Just like the name suggests, dyscalculia is a learning disability that makes it hard for kids to learn how to work out mathematical problems or grasp mathematical concepts.

- **Dysgraphia.** This learning disability is characterized by the inability to write. Children who have this disorder struggle to write or even form letters within a specified space.

- **Visual processing and auditory disorders.** A child who has these sensory disorders often struggles to understand language despite the fact that their senses of vision and hearing are normal.

- **Nonverbal Disabilities. These are typical neurological disorders, which often lead to difficulties in intuition, organization, spatial relations, and evaluation.**

What is the Connection Between Learning Difficulties and ADHD?

Dyslexia is the most common learning disorder in children. Research indicates that 15 to 20% of kids who have ADHD also suffer from a reading disability which is twice the average. In addition, impairments in the social, emotional, and academic areas of functioning are worse when a kid is affected by both ADHD and a learning difficulty. In the event that a kid is affected by a specific learning difficulty, there is a need to distinguish it from the attention and behavioral aspects of ADHD.

Tips to Overcome Learning Difficulties and ADHD

Since the possibility of a child with ADHD to also have a learning disability is high, there is a need for both disorders to be treated. The two disorders should be concurrently treated to attain the most desired outcome. For instance, if a child is being treated for ADHD, chances are high that their learning disability will persist. Likewise, if they are receiving assistance to treat their learning difficulty, the desired outcome possibly won't be attained if their problems of a lack of focus and impulsivity aren't addressed.

Generally, ADHD kids qualify to receive specialized education as stipulated by the Individuals with Disabilities Education Act.

Children who have ADHD, or any learning disability, are legally entitled to, and can benefit from an individualized education program that is designed to address their learning needs. Therefore, parents, guidance counselors, and teachers ought to work in tandem to form an IEP (individualized education program) before kids start school. The program needs to be regularly updated to accommodate the kids' emerging educational needs. In as much as neither learning disabilities nor ADHD can fully be cured, a kid can still live with the disorders and have a happy and successful life.

ADHD with Autism Spectrum Disorder in a Child and an Adult

Autism Spectrum Disorder (ASD) is a mental condition which makes the interaction and communication with others difficult. Kids and adults who have autism often face significant challenges. Typical symptoms that they exhibit can be: an inability to understand others' feelings, poor communication skills, delays in motor skills, poor understanding of abstract language uses such as conversation and humor, obsessive interest in certain information or items, and strong reaction to senses and stimuli.

On the other hand, ADHD is characterized by difficulties in paying attention, sitting still, and the tendency to act impulsively. The fourth edition of DSM-IV stipulated that both ADHD and ASD can't be co-diagnosed. However, DSM-5 recognized that the two disorders are interrelated and that both adults and kids can be affected concurrently by the two. Recently, DSM-5 was changed to eliminate the exclusion of the dual diagnosis of both ASD and ADHD.

Studies indicate that up to 29% of ASD kids aged between 4 and 8 years also exhibit some of the most common symptoms of ADHD. Moreover, adults and kids who have comorbid ADHD and ASD have significantly lower cognitive functioning, severe social impairment, and significant delays in adaptive functioning compared to children and adults who have ASD only. This shows that the presence of ADHD in kids and adults who have ASD greatly complicate their learning and understanding. Parents and family members of children and adults who have both conditions also report that those affected tend to have repetitive and stereotypical behaviors compared to those who either have ADHD or ASD alone.

Generally, behaviors that are associated with ASD tend to look like ADHD. This is why most of the symptoms of ASD and ADHD overlap. Kids and adults who suffer from ASD also have symptoms that typify ADHD. These include social awkwardness, an inability to stay calm, and impulsivity. Nevertheless, ADHD in its purest form isn't part of ASD.

What is the Difference Between ADHD and Autism?

Generally, ADHD is characterized by hyperactivity, inattention, and impulsivity. Therefore, the disorder inherently causes problems with executive function and self-regulation. On the other hand, Autism Spectrum Disorders are a continuum of disorders that include Asperger's syndrome, pervasive developmental disorder, and autism. These disorders are typified by problems when it comes to communication, social interactions, and repetitive mannerisms.

Children and adults who have autism don't intuitively

understand some of the aspects of the social world that exists around them. As a result, their social development, which is mirrored in their communication and interaction abilities, is greatly delayed. Besides this, these individuals exhibit specific symptoms including poor gesture language and limited imaginative play.

Even though the inherent components of both ASD and ADHD differ, there are a number of overlaps as far as the symptoms of the two disorders are concerned. The main trick as far as distinguishing the two conditions apart, is determining the exact developmental building block or executive function that is missing and thus causing the symptom. Generally, those battling with ADHD may struggle socially. With ADHD alone, proof of early social development, such as turn-taking play, responding to names, imaginative play, and gesture language usually remains intact. Traits such as displaying facial expressions, empathy, and humor also remain unaffected. When these traits are lacking, it is an indicator that an individual could be autistic. Kids and adults who have ADHD may not have the patience to wait in line but, they understand the concept. They also may not have the ability to respond when called as a result of inattention, but even so, they still remain socially engaged besides recognizing their names.

Diagnosing ASD and ADHD

If both ASD and ADHD are suspected in adults or children, it is advisable that a diagnosis is undertaken by a specialist who is familiar with the two disorders. A thorough examination should be done with the aim of defining the strengths and weaknesses of the affected individuals. Various tests should be carried out to document ADHD and ASD symptoms so that a clear distinction between the two can be made. Tests alone aren't sufficient since the evaluation of both autism and ADHD is a clinical skill, which is based heavily on getting to understand those who are affected by seeking a comprehensive picture of their lives and interactions in the real world. This will give the specialist an insight into the child's/adult's conversational and social skill, as well as their daily living or play skills.

Diagnosing ADHD and ASD can be a fluid and ongoing process rather than a one-off procedure. This is because those affected may initially exhibit ASD-like symptoms only for them to exhibit ADHD symptoms later on. You have to keep in mind the fact that, for people who have co-existing ASD and ADHD, treating either of the conditions first is a means to an end, which is treating the other. Few patients who have both ASD and ADHD succeed in life without medication.

Tips to Overcome ASD and ADHD Comorbidity

Just like it is the case with ADHD and learning difficulties, ADHD and ASD ought to be treated concurrently. Generally, the interventions used for both ASD and ADHD can help professionals make the most accurate diagnosis. For instance, ADHD medication can help quell the symptoms of the disorder and, in the process, make ASD symptoms clearer. For ADHD, there is substantial proof in favor of the use of medication and therapy to manage symptoms. For autism alone, there are medications that can help minimize specific symptoms, such as obsessive behavior. In either case, the underlying condition won't be treated; only their symptoms.

Non-medical interventions can also be used to help individuals who are suspected of having both ASD and ADHD before they receive a definite diagnosis. If those affected are experiencing ongoing social challenges, for instance, most of the interventions that will be used will be similar. This may include behavioral therapy to help them develop their social skills. To overcome the conditions, counseling and assistance ought to be offered to help those who are affected improve their social and organizational skills. Therapy will also help them grasp whatever gaps that exist between them and society. Other non-medical interventions, such as speech therapy, occupational therapy, parental training, and educational interventions, should also be explored.

ADHD With Anxiety

Anxiety often accompanies ADHD. Chances are high that if someone has been diagnosed with ADHD, they will also suffer from anxiety. Sometimes, anxiety is masked by the more prominent symptoms of ADHD. Nearly half of adults who have ADHD and 30% of kids with ADHD also suffer from an anxiety disorder. Typically, it is difficult to recognize even the most common symptoms of anxiety if you have ADHD. The behavioral disorder is a lifelong condition, which tends to mask other comorbid conditions that accompany it.

ADHD may make you feel uneasy, distressed, and excessively frightened in regular or benign circumstances. Those who have an anxiety disorder may exhibit symptoms that are so severe to the extent that their daily activities including work and study get compromised. In addition, they find it difficult to enjoy their social interactions and relationships. The inherent symptoms of an anxiety disorder differ from those of ADHD.

Primarily, ADHD symptoms involve issues pertaining to concentration and focus. On the other hand, anxiety symptoms involve issues that touch on nervousness and fear.

Each of these conditions has its own unique symptoms, with some crossing over to the other. This may make it hard for someone to tell the difference between the two disorders. Just like individuals who are battling with ADHD, those who suffer from an anxiety disorder tend to feel restless all the time, something that renders them unable to relax. Symptoms that are common in individuals suffering from an anxiety disorder alone include a chronic feeling of worry, fear without an obvious or plausible cause, irritability, insomnia, headaches or belly aches, and the fear of trying new things. Some of these symptoms are exhibited by individuals suffering from the various types of ADHD. For instance, children who have hyperactive-impulsive ADHD often have trouble sleeping. Likewise, inattentive type ADHD is sometimes exhibited by the fear of trying new things, especially those that seem to demand mental effort.

Differentiating Between Anxiety and ADHD

Even though a professional assessment is necessary to diagnose whether an individual is battling with both anxiety and ADHD, family members can easily tell the dissimilarities between the two conditions. The secret lies in watching how symptoms of the disorders play out over time. In case you are suffering from anxiety disorder, you may find it difficult to concentrate in circumstances that make you feel anxious. Conversely, those who have ADHD often find it difficult to concentrate most of the time regardless of the situation that they are in.

If you are battling with both ADHD and anxiety disorder, it's likely that the symptoms of both behavioral disorders will seem more extreme. For instance, anxiety may make it even harder for individuals who have ADHD to follow instructions or follow through tasks to the end.

In as much as comorbidity exists between these disorders, it isn't clear why there is a link between anxiety and ADHD. Researchers are yet to pinpoint what exactly causes the two disorders. To some extent, genetics may be responsible for these conditions, and may also lead to comorbidity. Often after ADHD has been diagnosed, anxiety typically sets in, particularly among adults because the condition gives them a lot to worry about. ADHD often causes individuals to utter inappropriate or offensive words without meaning to. In the process, they start worrying about their next move because they fear it might lead to offending others, and even with the law. Worrying too much about what might happen can lead to an anxiety disorder.

What is the Connection Between Anxiety and ADHD?

Most people who are diagnosed with ADHD tend to struggle with time-management skills, organizational skills, and working memory. This makes it hard for them to follow even the simplest of routines or complete long-term tasks. The ridicule that they receive for failing to undertake simple tasks often leads to chronic stress and worry. Children and adults who are suffering from ADHD also end up having problems with emotional regulation. In most cases, they become flooded with both positive and negative emotions, which are often difficult to manage. Ultimately, they end up struggling to make sense of their thoughts, and they also tend to get trapped in a web of anxious and negative thinking.

Since anxiety symptoms tend to mimic ADHD symptoms in both kids and adults, it is easy for a misdiagnosis to occur. This highlights the importance of ensuring that an accurate diagnosis is made via a thorough examination by a neuropsychologist. Anxiety may look like ADHD among kids. Therefore, it is advisable to have a kid assessed by a professional so that the best course of treatment is determined. In as much as the symptoms of ADHD and anxiety may overlap, you should take note of the fact that anxious children tend to exhibit more perfectionist behaviors without worrying about interacting with others. On the other hand, kids who have ADHD tend to struggle with organization and impulse control.

Diagnosis shouldn't be a one-off process. A complete neuropsychological assessment, including a classroom evaluation for kids, will help the specialist determine whether the child's behavior is entrenched in anxiety, ADHD, or a combination of the two disorders.

Tips to Overcome ADHD and Anxiety Disorder Comorbidity

If an individual is displaying symptoms of both anxiety and ADHD, it is advisable to treat both disorders. Treatment needs to be done by a mental health professional. Here are some tips for overcoming ADHD and anxiety disorder:

Understand Your Triggers

Usually, the symptoms of ADHD and anxiety are triggered by specific circumstances. These may include simple situations such as being asked to speak in public. It is advisable to identify situations that trigger anxiety and the symptoms of

ADHD. Once these triggers have been identified, one should work with a mental health professional to establish ways of dealing with the symptoms and anxiety, when faced with these situations. For instance, preparing notes to practice a presentation can go a long way in helping someone feel less anxious when speaking in front of an audience.

To manage anxiety in kids, it is also recommended to identify the exact stressors that make them feel anxious. This will help them learn how to foretell anxiety-inducing situations and as a result, he/she will be able to handle the symptoms as they occur.

Get Ample Rest

Tiredness and insufficient sleep increase the risk of feeling anxious. To counter sleep-induced anxiety, it is advisable that an individual sleeps for 7 to 8 hours per night. If someone has trouble falling asleep due to hyperactivity, meditating before bedtime to calm the mind will help. In addition, one should try going to bed and waking up at the same time each day.

In cases where medication is being taken for ADHD or anxiety, chances are high that it could be affecting sleep. In this case, an additional sleep aid, albeit temporarily, may be required. Avoid taking additional anxiety or sleep medication without consulting a doctor since it can make ADHD or anxiety symptoms even worse. Besides having sufficient sleep and rest, it is also good to exercise regularly.

Create a Schedule

If someone is suffering from ADHD, the completion of tasks may be a tall order. In most people, this makes their anxiety even worse. To avoid such a situation, it is advisable that you to create a schedule that will guide important and daily activities. Sticking to this schedule will help in their completion, without having to forget any. If ADHD exists, a person should avoid burdening or stressing themselves out about completing their tasks within schedule. Instead, they should expect for each task to take longer than the time allocated towards it. Setting unrealistic goals will only but worsen the anxiety.

Keep a Journal

There is no better way of suppressing anxiety than writing down what you feel about it. Writing a journal is one of the best ways of doing this since it clears your mind, besides enabling you to focus on what you are doing at that particular point. In addition, a journal makes you more committed towards your treatment, particularly if you develop the habit of going through it. To keep a journal, you must feel comfortable enough to write down whatever is on your mind at any particular time. This will help you pinpoint any issues that you would ultimately want to discuss with your therapist or doctor during your next visit.

Practice Thought Stopping

Thought stopping can be used to manage anxiety, especially within children. Generally, ADHD kids who also suffer from anxiety struggle with thought flooding. The anxious thoughts that flood their mind all at once often overwhelm them. Recovering from this is difficult because of the intricate pattern of anxious thinking. To prevent this situation, the children should be taught to practice thought stopping. During their calmest moments, have the kids practice telling themselves, "No brain, stop saying that to me. I can handle this." When kids learn to "talk back" to whatever is worrying them, it becomes easy for them to replace their anxious thoughts with more positive ones. It similarly becomes easy for them to interrupt the worry cycle whenever it creeps up, and to reset themselves accordingly. This also applies to adults who are battling ADHD and anxiety.

Deep Breathing

Breathing deeply is a tested and proven strategy for fighting anxiety, both in children and adults. Deep breathing not only slows down your heart-beat but also helps to relieve muscle tension. When individuals suffering from ADHD learn to deep breathe whenever worrying thoughts come up, they gain the ability to stay relaxed, thus dispelling such thoughts. With time, they develop the ability to handle their anxious thoughts accordingly and replace negative and anxious thinking with peaceful thinking.

Psychotherapy

Psychotherapy is one strategy that works for nearly all mental and behavioral disorders. If ADHD and comorbid anxiety impact daily life, career progression, and social interactions, psychotherapy from a mental health professional can really help. Through psychotherapy, ADHD kids and adults who are also suffering from anxiety will be able to manage their emotions. Besides this, they will develop the ability to identify stressors and anxiety triggers.

ADHD With Depression

ADHD and depression often go hand in hand since they tend to co-exist at the same time. Whereas ADHD affects an individual's ability to focus, depression is more than an infrequent case of the blues. This condition is characterized by a deep feeling of despair and sadness, which may last up to two weeks at a time. Depression may make it hard for you to attend to your daily duties or even fall asleep. Up to 30% of kids who have ADHD also suffer from a serious mood disorder. In addition, more than half of individuals who have ADHD get treated for depression at some point.

What is the Link Between ADHD and Depression?

Some of the most prominent symptoms of depression and ADHD are similar. This may make it hard to diagnose the conditions and treat them accordingly. For instance, those suffering from ADHD or depression may also have trouble with focus. If you take medication to aid with the ADHD symptom, your sleep or appetite is likely to be affected. Needless to say, these can also be symptoms of depression. In kids, irritability and hyperactivity are symptoms of ADHD as well as depression.

ADHD can also cause depression, especially in instances when those who are affected have trouble managing their symptoms. For instance, kids may have trouble when it comes to getting along with their peers at school or when playing. Likewise, adults may also have deep-seated issues at work. This can lead to a deep feeling of hopelessness, which is a common symptom of depression. In as much as medical practitioners cannot point out the exact cause of both depression and ADHD, the two conditions seem to be related to an individual's family history. Individuals who have ADHD or depression often have a family member who also has it.

Studies show that up to 70% of individuals suffering from ADHD have sought treatment for depression at some point. Teens who have ADHD are 10 times more likely to also suffer from depression, compared to those who do not have ADHD. Whereas boys are more likely to battle ADHD in their lives, girls have a higher risk of suffering from depression alongside

ADHD. Children who get diagnosed with ADHD when they are young are similarly at a higher risk of developing depression. Generally, individuals who have the inattentive type of ADHD are at a higher risk of depression compared to those battling with either the combination type of ADHD or the hyperactive-impulsive ADHD type.

Typically, individuals who have ADHD tend to experience mood swings that are triggered by certain events or circumstances. This is not the case among those suffering from depression, because their low mood may even last for months. Just like other mental disorders that are comorbid with ADHD, the main challenge when diagnosing depression and/or ADHD is the overlapping symptoms. These include feeling restless and experiencing difficulties in concentrating.

To compound the situation, most side effects of ADHD medications, such as insomnia and fatigue, tend to imitate depressive episodes. This highlights the significance of speaking to a psychiatrist, so that the exact cause of whatever symptoms are experienced, get pinpointed.

What Are the Distinguishing Symptoms Between ADHD and Depression?

Certain symptoms can be used to determine whether a patient is suffering from depression, ADHD, or both. Assessing these symptoms can go a long way in eliminating the confusion that exists as far as diagnosing ADHD and depression is concerned. Needless to say, differentiating these two disorders can be hard, owing to the fact that both lead to forgetfulness, mood problems, lack of motivation, and an inability to focus.

There are a number of subtle distinctions between symptoms

caused by depression and ADHD-induced symptoms.

- **Emotions.** ADHD can lead to low moods. These episodes are usually caused by specific setbacks. Moreover, the dark moods that ADHD patients may experience are usually transient in nature. On the other hand, the low mood issues that are linked to depression are pervasive and generally chronic in nature. They may last for weeks or months at a time. Unlike the low moods that are caused by ADHD which begin in childhood, depression doesn't usually develop until one reaches his/her teenage years.

- **Motivation.** When it comes to ADHD, it often seems impossible to complete any task. This comes about simply because those who are affected tend to dither without deciding which task they should tackle first. With depression, there is no uncertainty in the first place, patients are too lethargic to the extent that they cannot initiate any activity.

- **Sleep Problems.** With ADHD, individuals often experience problems once they get to bed. Due to their hyperactive nature, the minds of such individuals tend to simply refuse to "turn off." This contrasts sharply from people who are suffering from depression. They may instantly fall asleep as soon as they get to bed but they tend to sleep intermittently. Whenever they wake up repeatedly at night, their minds tend to be filled with anxious or negative thoughts.

Tips to Overcome Depression With ADHD

The most effective way of overcoming depression with ADHD is the use of medication, in order to quell the symptoms of each disorder. Even though these conditions tend to occur at the same time, one of them is likely to cause a greater impairment. You have to keep in mind the fact that even though problems caused by ADHD are real and serious, depression is a life-threatening disorder. Antidepressants that boost the level and performance of neurotransmitters can be used to remedy severe cases of ADHD with depression. In mild to moderate cases of depression with ADHD, an antidepressant can also be prescribed.

Most antidepressants are effective when used alongside ADHD stimulant and non-stimulant medication. Nearly half of individuals who take antidepressants to manage the symptoms of ADHD often end up achieving complete relief from symptoms of depression.

Apart from treatment, psychotherapy can effectively be used to treat depression with ADHD. The most efficient form of psychotherapy for use in this regard is cognitive behavioral therapy (CBT). This form of therapy mainly entails identifying the types of negative and anxious thoughts that individuals experience, and their frequency. Thereafter, work is done with the therapist to replace these self-destructive beliefs and thoughts with realistic thoughts. A negative thought such as "this is hard," will have to be replaced by a constructive one like, "Yes, this is hard, but I can manage." In as much as the difficulty of the task, you acknowledged, such a thought shows that the individual isn't wallowing in its difficulty. Instead, the direction is shifted to positive action for tackling that difficulty.

The objective of psychotherapy should be to minimize the intensity and frequency of not only the negative thoughts but also the symptoms of ADHD with depression.

You can also use meditation to treat depression that accompanies ADHD. For optimum results, sit in a quiet room with closed eyes. When doing this, focus solely on breathing while repeating a familiar word. It could be a spouse's name or a letter in the alphabet. Do this for 10-20 seconds every time a feeling of depressions sets in can go a long way in helping control ADHD and coexisting depression.

ADHD With Bipolar Disorder

It goes without saying that dealing with ADHD is a major challenge. Throw in bipolar disorder and it becomes even harder. It is difficult to distinguish between ADHD and bipolar disorder among kids and adults since both conditions have similar symptoms.

In its purest form, bipolar disorder is typified by mood swings between periods of extreme highs and lows. Bipolar in children is often a somewhat chronic mood deregulation characterized by a mix of elation, irritability, and depression.

There are certain symptoms that are present in kids suffering from both bipolar disorder and ADHD. These include a decreased need for sleep and high energy levels. In adults, bipolar disorder and ADHD tend to occur together. Between 15 and 17% of individuals who have bipolar disorder also suffer from ADHD. A clear distinction between the two conditions can be made owing to the fact that ADHD is characterized by the triad of impulsivity, restlessness, and distractibility. These symptoms must be present consistently and must also cause one form of impairment or another throughout an individual's life.

Bipolar disorder and ADHD can be differentiated by these pertinent factors:

- **Age of onset.** Generally, ADHD symptoms manifest themselves throughout an individual's lifetime. These symptoms ought to be present, though not necessarily impairing, by the age of 7. On its part, bipolar disorder can be present in preteens but even so, symptoms of the disorder tend to be so rare that researchers say it doesn't occur.

- **Consistency of symptoms and impairment.** ADHD remains present even when its symptoms seem to subside. On the other hand, bipolar disorder often occurs in intermittent episodes that are more or less determined by mood levels.

- **Triggered mood instability.** Individuals who have ADHD tend to be passionate, and have strong and emotional reactions to events happening around them. Whatever triggers the mood shifts with ADHD is different from what triggers the mood shifts in bipolar disorder. Happy circumstances in the lives of ADHD individuals tend to result in equally happy and elated states of mood. Likewise, unhappy circumstances resulting from rejection and criticism also result in a low mood.

Managing ADHD With Bipolar Disorder

At some point in our lives, we all are forced to cope with anger, anxiety, and impatience. Nevertheless, ADHD that is comorbid with bipolar disorder tends to magnify these emotions. In extreme cases, ever-changing moods can greatly interfere with careers, social interactions, and relationships. To cope with ADHD and bipolar, one should schedule appropriate times to vent, besides learning to take control of hyper-focus. Also, exercising more often will help removes negative energy.

Psychotherapy is often used alongside medical intervention to manage ADHD and bipolar disorder among kids and adults. You have to keep in mind the fact that even though medication alleviates some of the symptoms of ADHD and bipolar, individuals ought to make a deliberate effort to sign up for both individual therapy and psycho-education sessions. Psychotherapy classes typically entail teaching patients how to embrace their condition without feeling bitter about the impact that it might have had on their lives.

ADHD patients who are also finding it hard to complete tasks should also look to break them down into smaller portions. The completion of individual mini-tasks will give them a sense of accomplishment. What's more, it is advisable that adult ADHD individuals learn as much as they can about the disorder, since it will put them in a good position to face it.

Generally, a behavioral disorder affects job performance in various ways. If you cannot sit still during meetings, or if you have difficulties staying focused and organized, it will be hard for you to stay in one job for a substantial amount of time. Typically, individuals battling with ADHD and bipolar may have trouble with working memory, attention, verbal fluency, and mental processing. These qualities are generally referred to as executive-function abilities, and they come in handy at the workplace. Within the work environment, it is easy for you to get depressed or have low self-esteem if you have difficulties completing your tasks within schedules or beating simple deadlines. This may make your situation even worse.

The success of psychotherapy sessions for ADHD adults who also have bipolar starts with them remembering minor routines and keeping to the appointment time with the therapist. This is a step in the right direction, and will help them learn how to keep subsequent appointments with the therapist, and any other people that they are to meet in the future. Therapy for ADHD adults is done to help them know how best they can manage their condition. It similarly helps them learn how to change whatever long-standing poor self-image they might have. They do so by examining their experiences with the disorder in years gone by, and how to avoid the not-so-good ones.

Conclusion

ADHD is one of the most misunderstood behavioral disorders. Lots of myths and misconceptions exist pertaining to the disorder. In addition, it remains largely undetected in many people owing to the fact that its symptoms overlap with those of other mental disorders. There are also many myths and misconceptions about ADHD, something that has created confusion as what the condition really is, what causes it, and how it can be treated. Since ADHD affects many people, there is a need to raise awareness about it so that some of the misconceptions can be addressed.

Lastly, if you enjoyed this book I ask that you please take the time to review it on Audible.com. Your honest feedback would be greatly appreciated.

Thank you.

Now, I would like to share with you a free sneak peek to another one of my books that I think you will really enjoy. The book is called "Cognitive Behavioral Therapy (CBT): A Practical Guide to Free Yourself" Published by Lawrence M. Satterfield and Jason Wallace.

It's A Practical Guide to Learn the Most Effective CBT and DBT Techniques to Overcome Anxiety, Depression and Insomnia. You will also learn Exercises that will help you to Retrain your Brain and become more self-aware.

Enjoy!

The Mind with Cognitive Behavioral Therapy

will dig deeper into the practices of CBT and how you can benefit from them.

Firstly, it's important to understand how your brain responds to cognitive behavioral therapy. There have been some amazing studies on the matter. Not only does CBT affect your mind and the way you think, but it can also even affect how your brain operates as a biological function.

A group of researchers from universities in Sweden such as Linköping University decided to get together and study cognitive behavioral therapy. They did this because we have long known that the brain is incredibly adaptable. Some studies have even shown that activities such as video games and juggling can affect the volume of your brain.

To study how CBT affects the brain, the researchers conducted a study on a group of people by having them participate in cognitive behavioral therapy through the internet. One of the most common mental illnesses was the focus of this study. This illness is social anxiety disorder and affects an estimated fifteen million people within America.

Magnetic resonance imaging, commonly referred to as MRI, was conducted on all the participants both at the beginning and end of their CBT treatment. This study is amazing because not only do we have studies proving the mental effects of CBT, but this one is even looking at the biological effects.

In the initial brain scans, it was found that people with social anxiety disorder have an altered brain volume and the activity in a portion of their brain is increased. This portion of the brain is the amygdala, which is used primarily to make decisions, process memories, and emotional responses. It's easy to imagine how these changes could affect our mental state.

It may seem as if this biological function is out of our control, but this study proves otherwise. In fact, the study found that when the participants with social anxiety disorder completed nine weeks of CBT through the internet, their brains improved. These people experienced a reduction in brain volume and a decrease in the activity of the amygdala. The patients whose anxiety improved the most also experienced the greatest decrease in brain volume and amygdala activity.

This study proves the power of cognitive behavioral therapy. It isn't simply a false sense of positive thinking that some people may assume. Rather, it creates a real change in how you perceive the world, your reactions, your mood, and yes, even your brain.

What about people like Mary who suffers from debilitating depression? I have good news. Cognitive behavioral therapy has had great success on people living with depression. The results are amazing. CBT has been shown to be twice as effective as antidepressants in preventing depressive relapses.

The study which proved this was hoping to find the effects of both antidepressants and CBT on depressed people. While the researchers hypothesized that both treatments would treat depression similarly, they were surprised by the results.

Throughout treatment with some participants on antidepressants and others practicing cognitive behavioral therapy, the researchers would scan their brains with an MRI.

They were soon surprised to find that antidepressants and CBT impact completely different areas of the brain for people with depression. Antidepressants would reduce the activity in the emotional center of the brain known as the limbic system. Surprisingly, CBT helped to calm the area of the brain which is responsible for our reasoning, the cortex.

This means that while antidepressants reduce our emotions, CBT can actively help us to process them in a more proactive and healthy manner. This explains why CBT is much more effective in the long run and less likely to result in a depressive relapse down the road.

Post-traumatic stress disorder, often simply referred to as PTSD is a common condition which people suffer from after undergoing a traumatic event. Most people only consider veterans who went to war having PTSD. However, there are many other people who live every day with this condition. For instance, people who have undergone painful surgeries, those who have been in accidents, people who have lost someone close to them, and sexual assault victims. The symptoms of PTSD vary from person to person, but a few of the symptoms include:

- Flashbacks reliving a traumatic experience.
- Nightmares.
- Avoiding events, places, or objects that remind a person of the traumatic experience.
- Feeling tense, on edge, and easily startled.
- Experiencing angry outbursts.
- Having difficulty sleeping.
- Difficulty remembering or recalling the traumatic event.

- Guilt, blame, or other negative thoughts towards yourself.
- Loss of interest in your daily life and enjoyable activities.

There is much more, but these are some of the most common symptoms of PTSD. If you suspect you may have PTSD, please talk with a psychologist or psychiatrist and they can walk you through it. It is always recommended to get help from a trained professional who can personalize your care and treatment plan. However, this book can help alongside your doctor during your journey towards healing.

One study showing the effects of cognitive behavioral therapy was conducted with the participation of one-hundred children who were suffering from PTSD after being sexually assaulted. They had the children go into therapy, some with their mothers present and others with solely the therapist. Their condition was checked at regular intervals to see how the children were healing from the trauma.

The children completed tests both before, during, and after the treatment periods. After the original cognitive behavioral therapy, the children's tests scores improved significantly. These continued to improve over the following two years. This suggests that CBT is a successful treatment option for long-term improvement and care.

But in order to receive these benefits, it is important to understand in-depth how to utilize cognitive behavioral therapy. This therapy is a powerful tool and if you understand its basis and how to follow it through, you can experience amazing benefits.

While cognitive behavioral therapy involves some positive thinking, there is more to it than that. In fact, if you tell a person who is depressed, anxious, stressed, or suffering from trauma simply "just think positively," it will only cause them further stress. This is because positive thoughts alone are not enough to cause lasting change. When a person tries this and it doesn't work, they are likely to feel frustrated. This down-spiral further increases negative thoughts.

Instead, it is important to practice using your mind as a tool over your mood. This will help you to consider all the information you have access to from various angles. If you are able to consider a situation (whether negative or positive) from all sides, then you can find a new understanding and solutions to your problems.

A good example of this is Lydia. If she simply told herself "I won't have anxiety when I see the neighbor's dog. I'm perfectly fine," she would be unrealistic and wouldn't be prepared for the anxiety she is likely to face once she sees the dog. Once she begins to feel anxiety upon seeing the dog, Lydia may end up feeling like a failure. Even a small amount of anxiety will make her feel as if there is no point to positive thinking.

Instead, Lydia will do better if she studies the situation from all sides and then decides on a solution for how to react if she becomes anxious. She can then think positively trusting in herself and her plan to help get her through coming across dogs. This is more successful because if we only allow false positive thoughts, then we will be unprepared for difficult situations.

Identifying your thoughts and then analyzing, testing, considering alternatives, and using your mind over your mood are important aspects of CBT. Although it is equally important to make behavioral changes along with these, it is important to keep in mind that cognitive behavioral therapy is consists of many components. Just like the inner pieces of a clock, CBT is only successful when all of the parts are working together.

Work on identifying your thoughts and analyzing them, thinking more positively, coming up with plans to reduce anxiety, and more. But also makes changes in your life. These changes will vary from person to person.

Rather than avoiding all dogs, Lydia could try acclimating to friendly small dogs until she feels comfortable. This will help her overcome her fear overtime and learn how to better manage her anxiety.

Mary needs to make a point of communicating with friends and spending time doing enjoyable activities. Her depression may make her feel like doing nothing but lying in bed and staring at the ceiling. But in order to improve the depression, she needs to get back out into life.

With Matt's alcoholism, he shouldn't keep alcohol around the house or go to bars. Instead, he needs to make a goal of becoming sober and attend regular meetings for alcoholics.

Likewise, if someone is being abused, they shouldn't simply "think happy thoughts" and become more submissive to their oppressor. Instead, their focus should be on finding a safe way to escape the abusive situation.

Now that you understand that this process is not solely about a false and short lasting positive thinking, it is time to address our negative thought processes. These thoughts control our actions in many ways. Maybe you were too scared to follow the career of your dreams because you might fail. Perhaps you become so overwhelmed that you procrastinate constantly. Or maybe you begin binge eating because you ate a single cookie and feel like a failure so what even is the point? All of these negative thoughts and more are damaging. Over time, they not only prevent us from attaining our goals and the life we desire, but they also will increasingly affect our mental health.

This is because of our negative thoughts and circumstances will accumulate. This shows in Lydia's story, where her trauma of dogs didn't surface until after she had been through a stressful divorce, move, and promotion. After all of the negative thoughts and emotions of the past year accumulated, she was unable to handle the anxiety and it manifested by bringing back her childhood trauma.

These thoughts can also combine in ways that make us think more negatively of ourselves such as in Matt's case, or as if there is no point in doing anything, like with Mary.

It is important to recognize all of your negative thoughts and learn to analyze and test them and then overcome them. But to do that, first, you need to know how to recognize them. There are ten main types of negative thoughts. Many people will experience most, if not all of these from time to time. But people often fall into centering on one or two types of negative thoughts.

These include:

1. Focusing on the Negative: *"Everything always goes wrong, life is just one disappointment after another."*

2. Negative Labeling of Yourself: *"I'm a terrible person and a failure. If people knew who I really was, they would leave me."*

3. Perfectionism: *"I have to do everything perfectly, otherwise I am a failure. I can't let anyone see anything of mine unless it's perfect."*

4. Constant Approval Needed: *"I have to make everyone like me. That's the only way I can be happy."*

5. Worst Case Scenario: *"Everything is going to be a disaster. It can't go well. I'm doomed."*

6. Ignoring the Present: *"I'll take care of myself later. For now, I have a list of things to accomplish."*

7. Other People Should Do What I Think: *"My friend shouldn't be posting so many photos of her boyfriend on social media. My adult daughter shouldn't be pursuing that career. That stranger shouldn't be wearing that, it's unflattering."*

8. Mind Reader: *"Other people must hate me, otherwise they wouldn't behave that way."*

9. Living in the Past: *"I'm miserable. I'm going to lay here and think about what happened to make me feel this way."*

10. Glass Half Empty: *"I don't trust people who are happy. If anything good ever happens in my life, then it is all going to be destroyed."*

The thoughts will vary from person to person depending on their situation. But most people will fit into at least one or two of these categories. After we figure out how we think, we can begin to counteract it. To do this, we start by finding the deceptions within those thought patterns.

Keep a little notebook with you or simply use a smartphone and keep track of your negative thoughts. You want a list that resembles sections titled:

- Situation
- Mood
- Automatic Thoughts or Images
- Evidence that Supports my Thoughts

- Evidence that Disproves my Thoughts
- Alternative Healthy Thoughts
- New Mood

When creating this list, you should use the four W's to help you. This means always fill out who, what, when, and where. You want to be specific, because if you simply state that it was happening "all day," then you are unable to target the cause behind the feelings. But if you know that you felt this way at 8:30 am when you were on your way to work, this narrows things down greatly.

Under the mood column, write any and all of the moods you were feeling at the time. You may have been feeling overwhelmed, depressed, anxious, sad, hurt, nervous, angry, or other emotions. When listing these, it is beneficial to rate them on a score of zero to one-hundred. These allow people who experience panic or anxiety attacks to log the severity.

Under the automatic thoughts or images, write any of the thoughts that were going through your head at the time. Taking the example from a moment ago, imagine that the thoughts running through your mind on the way to work that triggered this were *"I'm going to be late," "They'll fire me and then I won't have a job,"* and *"I'm worthless"*. If these thoughts were running through your head, you would write them down in this column and then analyze them in the following columns.

Next, tie together the columns for automatic thoughts and mood together on a rating of zero to one-hundred. For each thought, rate how it made you feel. Did the thought of being late makes you twenty percent anxious? The thought of being fired and without a job eighty percent scared? The thought of being worthless ninety percent depressed? By ranking the emotions tied to each of these thoughts, you can learn to better recognize damaging thoughts and proceed to overcome them.

The following step is one of the most important in this method and that is analyzing the evidence on whether or not your feelings are true or false. This can help us learn to identify what is a fact rather than our interpretation of a situation. There are many questions you can ask yourself to analyze these thoughts, but in the example we have been exploring, you might ask "Do I know I won't make it to work on time," "Are they likely to fire someone for being late once," "am I blaming myself for something out of my control," "When I'm not feeling this way, what do I think of this situation," "Are there any positives about myself that I am ignoring", and "If my best friend knew how I was feeling, what would they say?"

After analyzing the thought, you can fill in the alternative healthy thought section. Here, if you found that your thoughts weren't true, then you could fill in a more accurate thought. This might be "I haven't been late this year and my boss loves me, they are unlikely to fire me. I know I'm not worthless, every person has value and I have learned to be kind and compassionate. I am a valuable person"

If your thoughts were partially true, take the new information to write a more balanced view. For instance "my boss won't be happy, but I doubt I will be without a job. I may have slept through my alarm this morning, but that doesn't negate my intrinsic worth as a human being. I can take steps to wake up on time in the future."

After you analyze your thoughts and create new healthier and more balanced thoughts, you can rate how the new thoughts make you feel on a level of zero to one-hundred like you did with the original thought.

While this forum will change moment by moment for any given person, depending on the situations they are going through, let's look at what it might look like if Mary and Matt filled out this forum.

Mary:

- **Situation:**
  Didn't answer the phone when a friend called at noon.

- **Mood:**
  Depressed ninety percent, anxious thirty percent, worthlessness fifty percent.

- **Automatic Thoughts or Images:**
  "I can't be close to people. If I am, they'll die and I'll lose them," "I'm bad luck to have around," "Why am I even alive?"

- **Evidence that Supports my Thoughts:**
  My loved ones keep dying.

- **Evidence that Disproves my Thoughts:**
  Death is a part of life.
  My friends and pets were ill.
  I cared for them as best as I could do while they were alive.
  Their deaths were out of my hands.
  People aren't bad or good luck.
  Everyone is alive for a purpose.
  My friends care about me and want me around.

- **Alternative Healthy Thoughts:**
  "I'm sad that they died, but it wasn't my fault and I can't blame myself. My friends care about me and if I wasn't around, they would be sad."

- **New Mood:**
  Depressed forty percent, sad twenty percent, hopeful twenty percent.

As you can see, Mary may not feel all better, but she is working through her emotions. Her thoughts and mood are more stable now and she is reminded of why she is alive.

Now, let's look at Matt:

- **Situation:**
  His ex-girlfriend came by for a box of her stuff at 6 pm.

- **Mood:**
  Angry eighty percent, sad fifty percent.

- **Automatic Thoughts or Images:**
  "Why did she have to come by tonight when I was already having a bad day? She should have known it was too soon to see each other, now I miss her even more. This is her fault. If she had only forgiven me. I want a drink."

- **Evidence that Supports my Thoughts:**
  I apologized, she could have forgiven me.

- **Evidence that Disproves my Thoughts:**
  She needed her stuff and had a right to come get it. Even after the breakup, she was being kind and asked how I was doing.

  The breakup isn't her fault. She stuck with me for two years despite my drinking and anger. She doesn't have to forgive me and even if she has, that doesn't mean she is required to stay with me.

- **Alternative Healthy Thoughts:**

    "I'm sad that we broke up, but I hope she lives a happy life. Now that I am single, I can focus on bettering my own life, becoming sober, and controlling my temper. This is better for both of us in the long-run. A drink won't help me and I want to stay sober."

- **New Mood:**

    Sad fifteen percent, encouraged twenty percent, motivated fifty percent.

While Matt began the process as angry, as he worked through his feelings, whether they were true or false and developed a healthier alternative thought, he was able to work through his anger. This helped him to accept the breakup at the moment and encouraged him to stay sober. He may struggle with his anger and the breakup from time to time in the future, but if he continues to get through it in this healthy manner, then he can improve his life, learn to control his anger, and resist alcohol. Over time, the breakup will begin to hurt less.

It is important to retain awareness of your own mental state. To do this, try to fill out this forum regularly, especially whenever you notice your mood is low or your thoughts are destructive. But sometimes it can be hard to start because we are greatly lacking an awareness of our thoughts. This can be especially true when we have been living with a condition such as depression or anxiety for a long time. We become so accustomed to it that it turns into background noise. We need to learn to listen into this background noise so that we can tune it into a beautiful melody rather than a high-pitched static. Asking different questions based on our moods can help.

Generalized questions are a good place to start because you can ask them of yourself, no matter what your mood is. You may find it difficult to place a finger on exactly what you had been thinking of prior to a mood shift, but with some time, you will become an expert at realizing and recalling what is impacting your mood. After practice, many people will be able to place their finger on what upset them simply by answering these two questions:

- What was the last thing going through my mind before I noticed my mood shift?
- What memories or images was I experiencing?

The second question is regarding images and memories because many people find that their strongest mood shifts aren't a response to a specific thought. Rather, it was a response to a memory or image they thought of. For instance, for a split second, someone could remember a still image of a loved one in the hospital. If you have a lot going on in your life, it is easy to get distracted and not remember what triggered it, but the negative emotions remain. This is why it's important to learn to target and analyze what is affecting you.

After answering the generalized questions, you can answer some more specific mood-related questions.

When people are anxious, they often consider worst-case scenarios of what could happen in the near or distant future. We overestimate what could go wrong while simultaneously underestimating ourselves. When you find yourself anxious, scared, or nervous, then ask yourself *"what am I afraid might happen?"* and *"what is the worst that could happen?"*

If you find yourself depressed, it is easy to be self-critical or even hate yourself completely. In this case, it's easy to not just be critical about ourselves, but life in general as well. Therefore, if you are feeling depressed, sad, discouraged, or disappointed, I want you to ask yourself three questions.

"What does this mean about me?", "What does this mean about my future?", and *"What does this mean about life?"*

People often feel guilt or shame in conjunction with their actions even if they didn't do anything wrong. For instance, people can have survivor's guilt if someone close to them died yet they survived. There was nothing wrong with them surviving and they couldn't have saved the other person, yet they feel guilty. Though these feelings can, of course, have validity as well. If you got into a fight with your sibling, you could feel guilty for something you said. If you find yourself feeling this way, ask yourself *"Did I hurt someone, break a law/rule, not have done something I should have, or otherwise gone against my moral code?", "What does this mean about how others feel about me?", "What do I think or believe about myself?",* and *"What would other people think if they knew?"*

We can often feel angry, irritated, or resentful if we have felt as if someone has harmed us in some way. Even if the person wasn't unjust or mistreating us, we can often feel antsy from anger. It is important to distinguish whether or not this anger is justified. There is righteous anger. For instance, we can be angry when we learn of a child being abused. Non-righteous anger would be us getting angry that the cheeseburger that we ordered had pickles when we asked for no pickles. Sure, the person who made the cheeseburger made a mistake, but it is not something to get upset about if they are willing to fix it for us. If you are having anger related feelings, ask yourself *"What does this mean about other people?"* and *"What does this mean about how other people feel about me?"*

By asking yourself these questions, you will learn to recognize your emotions and the thoughts, memories, and images that trigger them. While what other people do and say can impact our emotions, remember that it is ultimately how we respond to those people that impact our long-term emotional state.

Occasionally, you may want to try looking over some of the other questions that aren't in your emotional category. For instance, if you are feeling anxious, you still may benefit by asking yourself the depression questions. Over time, you may even develop some of your own questions which you find is helping you to identify why you are feeling or reacting in specific ways.

Thank you, this preview is now over.

I hope you enjoyed this preview of my book Cognitive Behavioral Therapy (CBT).

Please make sure to check out the full book on Amazon.com

Thank you.